Orthopaedics for the Medical Student

Contributors

J. David Blaha, M.D.
Associate Professor of Orthopedic Surgery
Department of Orthopedic Surgery
West Virginia University School of Medicine
Morgantown, West Virginia

Charles M. Davis, M.D.
Clinical Professor of Orthopedic Surgery
Department of Orthopedic Surgery
West Virginia University School of Medicine
Morgantown, West Virginia

Eric T. Jones, M.D., Ph.D.
Associate Professor of Orthopedic Surgery
Department of Orthopedic Surgery
West Virginia University School of Medicine
Morgantown, West Virginia

David A. Labosky, M.D., Ph.D.
Associate Professor of Orthopedic Surgery
Department of Orthopedic Surgery
West Virginia University School of Medicine
Morgantown, West Virginia

Rudolf K. Lemperg, M.D., Ph.D.
Orthopedic Staff
Martinsburg City Hospital
Martinsburg, West Virginia
Formerly Professor of Orthopedic Surgery
Department of Orthopedic Surgery
West Virginia University School of Medicine
Morgantown, West Virginia

Justus C. Pickett, M.D.
Emeritus Professor of Orthopedic Surgery
Department of Orthopedic Surgery
West Virginia University School of Medicine
Morgantown, West Virginia

Eric L. Radin, M.D.
Professor and Chairman of Orthopedic Surgery
Department of Orthopedic Surgery
West Virginia University School of Medicine
Morgantown, West Virginia

Jamshid Tehranzadeh, M.D.
Associate Professor of Radiology
University of Miami
Miami, Florida
Formerly Associate Professor of Radiology and Orthopedic Surgery
Department of Orthopedic Surgery
West Virginia University School of Medicine
Morgantown, West Virginia

Andrea K. Faulkner
Formerly Editorial Associate
Department of Orthopedic Surgery
West Virginia University School of Medicine
Morgantown, West Virginia

ORTHOPAEDICS
for the Medical Student

Edited by

Eric L. Radin, M.D.
Department of Orthopedic Surgery
West Virginia University School of Medicine
Morgantown, West Virginia

With 8 contributors

J. B. Lippincott Company
Philadelphia
London Mexico City New York St. Louis São Paulo Sydney

Sponsoring Editor: Richard Winters
Manuscript Editor: Janet Greenwood
Indexer: Ann Cassar
Design Director: Tracy Baldwin
Design Coordinator: Anne O'Donnell
Production Supervisor: J. Corey Gray
Production Assistant: Charlene Catlett Squibb
Compositor: TAPSCO, Inc.
Printer/Binder: R. R. Donnelley

Copyright © 1987, by J. B. Lippincott Company. All rights reserved. No part of this book may be used or reproduced in any manner whatsoever without written permission except for brief quotations embodied in critical articles and reviews. Printed in the United States of America. For information write J. B. Lippincott Company, East Washington Square, Philadelphia, Pennsylvania 19105.

6 5 4 3 2 1

Library of Congress Cataloging-in-Publication Data

Orthopaedics for the medical student.

   Bibliography: p.
   Includes index.
   1. Orthopedia.   I. Radin, Eric L. [DNLM: 1. Orthopedics.   WE 168 07628]
RD731.078   1987   617'.3   86-10676
ISBN 0-397-50744-5

The authors and publisher have exerted every effort to ensure that drug selection and dosage set forth in this text are in accord with current recommendations and practice at the time of publication. However, in view of ongoing research, changes in government regulations, and the constant flow of information relating to drug therapy and drug reactions, the reader is urged to check the package insert for each drug for any change in indications and dosage and for added warnings and precautions. This is particularly important when the recommended agent is a new or infrequently employed drug.

Preface

Over the last 80 years, since the development of diagnostic x-ray, orthopaedics has grown beyond the application of brace and traction to become a recognized and highly respected field of medicine able to radically improve the quality of patients' lives. Although it has been more difficult to apply the principles of molecular biology to the calcified skeletal system than to soft tissue, today's orthopaedic diagnosis and treatment have a firm basis in musculoskeletal physiology and functional anatomy. Yet, despite these advances, the discipline remains in some instances incomplete and controversial. We acknowledge this but we also appreciate the fact that the beginning student has to start somewhere and that a hypothesis is a better learning aid than no explanation at all. For this reason, we have favored here a relatively dogmatic approach.

This brief volume is not intended to be a comprehensive overview of orthopaedics but rather an introduction to the principles that define sound orthopaedic practice. The section of selected readings allows the student to enter orthopaedic literature in an orderly fashion.

The text is based on the curriculum offered by the Department of Orthopedics at West Virginia University School of Medicine and is indebted to the suggestions of medical students who have rotated through the Department. As editor I wish to thank the contributors, present and former members of the Department, who frequently acted as a team rather than as individuals, making the unification of this material much easier. I will always be grateful to the secretaries of our department, particularly Sylvia Powley and Cassandra Watkins, who have struggled with this syllabus for many years with consummate skill and without complaint, and to my editorial associate, Cindy Weber, whose invaluable liaison with the publisher greatly facilitated the production of this volume.

Eric L. Radin, M.D.

Contents

Part One
Evaluation of the Orthopaedic Patient   *1*

  1 History and Physical and Radiographic Examinations   *3*
     Justus C. Pickett and Eric L. Radin

Part Two
Trauma   *7*

  2 Fractures and Dislocations   *9*
     Charles M. Davis

  3 Injuries of the Hand   *35*
     David A. Labosky

  4 Injuries of the Neck   *57*
     David A. Labosky

  5 Sports Injuries   *63*
     Eric L. Radin

Part Three
Adult Orthopaedic Problems   *75*

  6 Reaction of Bone to Tumors and Infections   *77*
     Rudolf K. Lemperg, Jamshid Tehranzadeh, and Eric L. Radin

  7 Arthritis and Arthrosis   *93*
     J. David Blaha and Eric L. Radin

  8 Pain in the Back and Leg   *113*
     Eric L. Radin and Jamshid Tehranzadeh

Part Four
Pediatric Orthopaedic Problems 129

9 Congenital and Developmental Conditions 131
   Eric T. Jones

10 The Limping Child 149
   Eric T. Jones

11 Scoliosis 161
   Eric T. Jones

Selected Readings 167

Glossary 171

Index 181

Part One

Evaluation of
the Orthopaedic Patient

Chapter 1

History and Physical and Radiographic Examinations

Justus C. Pickett and Eric L. Radin

History

As in all branches of medicine, as much as 80% of the diagnosis may be made on the basis of a careful medical history. Important details include onset and duration of the difficulty, character and location of the problem and, very important, the factors that tend to aggravate or alleviate the symptoms. Because the extremities are innervated dermatomically, they are frequently the site of referred pain, for example, pain in the leg from lumbosacral facet joint difficulties, pain in the knee from hip joint problems, and pain in the arm from cervical radiculitis. Thus, in orthopaedics the location of the pain may not be diagnostically reliable.

In considering the factors that influence symptoms, one can make a distinction between pain caused by inflammation and pain of a mechanical origin. Discomfort from edema around joints will be worse after rest (*e.g.,* morning stiffness), whereas pain from mechanical factors will be worse after activity (usually at the end of the day).

It is also important to note whether particular motions and activities result in symptoms and whether any functional impairment is experienced.

Although theoretically important, the character of pain is rarely diagnostic in practice. Frequently patients with worn-out joints will complain of burning pains, and patients with disc disease may not complain of toothachelike or other "neurogenic" type pain. Coughing and sneezing raise venous pressure and may aggravate any pain. Unfortunately, these symptoms do not contribute information helpful with a specific diagnosis.

Physical Examination

Localized tenderness is one of the most important signs for determining the anatomic location of a patient's musculoskeletal difficulty. With careful palpation one can differentiate between the joint and the periarticular areas or localize a spinous interspace that is causing the patient difficulty. Knowing the location of the ligamentous structures and palpating them carefully will usually allow one to distinguish tears of ligaments in the subcutaneous joints (particularly about the ankle) from fractures.

Swelling and Effusion

The elbow, wrist, hand, acromial and sternoclavicular joints, knee, ankle, and forefoot are subcutaneous and can be easily inspected for localized swelling. Joint effusions can be palpated in all joints except in the hip. An effusion of the shoulder should be sought anteriorly. A joint effusion is an indication that there is really something wrong in the joint or immediately adjacent to the synovial membrane; it is a finding that lends considerable seriousness to the diagnostic possibilities. Infections should always be considered in all age groups; one should look for local signs of inflammation (redness, heat, swelling).

Range of Motion

The examiner should carefully record, in degrees, the ranges of motion of the joints and, with the appendicular skeleton, compare right to left. With experience one can recognize the increased range of motion of infantile and growing joints and the limited range of motion associated with senescence. These must be distinguished from pathological losses of joint motion.

Examination should be carried out both passively (the examiner moving the segments) and actively (the patient moving the segments). When examining the passive range, one should proceed with care and not attempt to force motions. The patient's response to various positions can be very useful in determining the location of the pathology within the joint.

Presence of full passive range but splinting of the active range of motion suggests aggravation of the underlying pathology by muscle contraction; one example would be pain experienced with abduction of a shoulder with a subdeltoid bursitis. In such a situation, if one overcomes the guarding, one may abduct the shoulder passively, causing little discomfort.

Functional limitations of the musculoskeletal apparatus may frequently be neurogenic in origin; thus a complete neurologic evaluation (muscle strength, sensory and reflex testing) should also be undertaken.

Gross Deformity

Angular deformity, holding the body part in an abnormal position, and abnormal motions or gaits can be significant diagnostic indicators. For example, when a patient with acute low-back pain holds his trunk away from the side in which the pain is experienced, the difficulty is likely to be lateral to the nerve root. If a patient tilts toward the pain from a ruptured disc, the investigator should suspect that the pathology is medial to the involved nerve root.

When a patient is experiencing difficulty with the patellofemoral joint, the lower extremity should be examined for angular and rotatory abnormalities to see if the patella is tracking centrally down the intercondylar femoral groove. A patient with valgus deformities (knock-knees), for example, will tend to pull the kneecaps laterally when bending the knees, suggesting subluxation as a cause of the symptoms.

Radiographic Examination

Radiographic examination should be undertaken only when the history and physical examination suggest that the risk of radiation is worthwhile. Radiographic examination should not be used, except in the case of an unconscious injured patient, as a screening procedure for orthopaedic injury. Physical examination will suggest what parts need to be viewed. Because of the commonness of referred pain in the limbs, radiography should never be considered a substitute for a complete history and physical examination.

X-ray views must be biplanar for full visualization of the bones (see Fig. 2-3). Single views can be misleading, particularly in the cases of oblique fractures and dislocations.

Ligamentous integrity can be tested by checking for joint stability. Although this will not reveal partial tears of ligaments, it will distinguish complete ligamentous ruptures.

In the radiographic evaluation of injuries about the joints of young children, the inexperienced observer is well advised to compare films of involved joints with those of the respective uninvolved joints to avoid confusing the normal anatomy of the epiphyseal growth centers (particularly in the immature elbow) with injury. Anatomic osseous abnormality may sometimes be asymptomatic, as in the case of bipartite patellas. It may also be unilateral; in this instance diagnosis is dependent upon the knowledge of the special radiographic appearance of the abnormality, derived from experience.

Part Two

Trauma

Chapter 2

Fractures and Dislocations

Charles M. Davis

A fracture is a break in the structural integrity of bone and is usually associated with some degree of injury to the adjacent soft tissue. Dislocation is the disruption of a joint; subluxation is a partial dislocation.

The type and location of a fracture depend upon several biomechanical factors including the characteristics of the applied load tending to cause the fracture and the characteristics of the bone that cause it to resist fracture. Load characteristics include the direction of the applied force (tension, compression, bending, and torsion), the magnitude of the load, and the rate of load application. High-magnitude and high-velocity loads cause high energy to be imparted to bone, resulting in comminution of fracture and more extensive soft-tissue damage.

Resistance of bone to fracture is a factor of the geometry, structure, and material properties of the bone. Osteoporosis, a decrease in bone mass per unit volume, is an example of how a decrease in the material strength of bone predisposes it to fracture. The shape of a bone also influences its strength. The hollow, cylindrical shape of the long bones is efficient for resistance to fracture torsion or bending, using a minimal amount of tissue to most effect (Fig. 2-1). A defect in the integrity of a bone caused by a screw hole or erosion by tumor leads to a concentration of stress at those points, thereby increasing susceptibility to fracture (Fig. 2-2).

Fractures are caused by (1) abnormally high loads applied to normal bone, (2) normal loads applied to abnormal bone, and (3) low levels of repetitive cyclical loading of normal bone leading to structural fatigue. When normal loads cause fractures in abnormal bone, the term

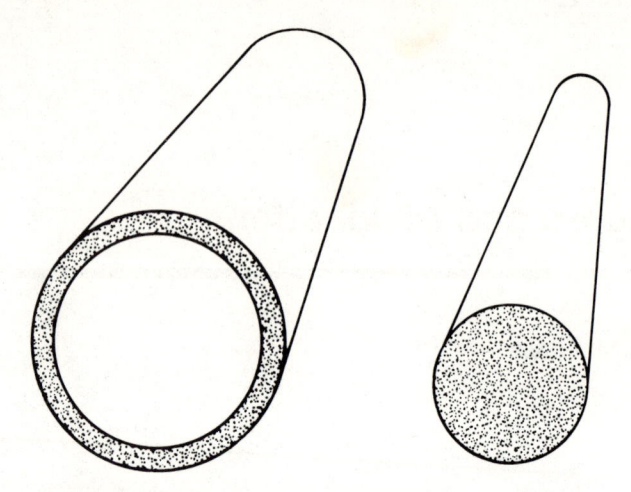

Figure 2-1. Even though both cylinders are made of equivalent amounts of material, the hollow cylinder on the left is several times stronger in torsion and bending than the solid cylinder on the right.

"pathological fracture" is used. Postmenopausal osteoporosis is the most common underlying condition predisposing to fracture. Carcinoma metastatic to bone is the next-most-common cause. Repetitive cyclical loading of bone can cause a painful stress or fatigue fracture, a condition frequently seen in runners.

Dislocation of a joint may or may not appear in conjunction with fracture of bone. In dislocations the soft tissues limiting joint excursion—that is, the joint capsule and ligaments—have been torn. Dislocations are extremely painful, sometimes even when the extremity is splinted. Blood vessels that supply the metaphysis of bones enter through the soft tissues near the joint. Dislocation puts these periarticular tissues on stretch or can tear them, cutting off the blood supply to the epiphysis. Loss of this blood supply can lead to osteonecrosis (bone death) or paralysis.

Clinical Features of Fractures and Dislocations

The diagnosis of severely displaced and angulated fractures or joint dislocations is easily made. Other injuries, however, may be difficult to diagnose without a careful history, physical and radiographic eval-

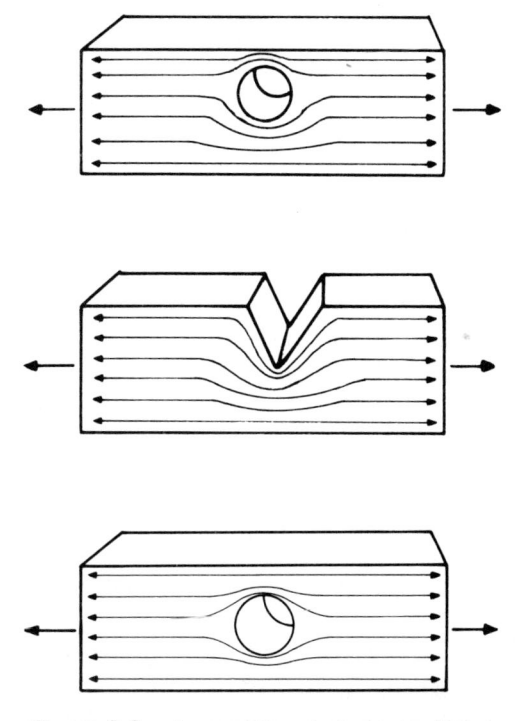

Figure 2-2. Any notch or hole concentrates stress. (After Radin EL, Simons SR, Rose RM, Paul JL: Practical Biomechanics for the Orthopedic Surgeon, p 51. New York, John Wiley & Sons, 1979)

uations, and a high index of suspicion. Such injuries might include undisplaced fracture of the scaphoid, impacted subcapital fractures of femoral neck, and undisplaced epiphyseal fractures. Suggestive signs and symptoms are listed below.

Pain. All fractures and dislocations cause some degree of pain in neurologically intact patients. The pain from fractures is usually well localized and is aggravated by attempts at motion. Occasionally the pain may be referred distally (*e.g.,* hip fracture causing knee pain) and thus lead to a difficult diagnosis. The major causes of pain after fracture or dislocation are unremitting muscle spasm (the body's mechanism to stabilize the disrupted segment) and reaction to local hemorrhage and edema.

Tenderness. Localized tenderness directly over bone is a fairly reliable sign of underlying fracture. This is usually a good way to differentiate a sprain from a fracture, but it is not always reliable.

Loss of Function. Functional loss can be caused by pain. Although functional loss may be present, it, like tenderness, is not a reliable sign.

Deformity. This is due primarily to malposition of fracture fragments of bones. Some fractures and dislocations result in a characteristic position of the extremity. Examples of this would be the shortening and external rotation of the lower extremity due to an intertrochanteric fracture of the femur and the shortening and internal rotation of the lower extremity due to a posteriorly dislocated hip.

Crepitus. This transmitted grating sound of fractured bone ends moving on each other is painful to elicit and should not be purposely sought.

Careful neurovascular examination is essential in evaluating patients with fractures or dislocations, since neurovascular injuries are frequently associated with fracture.

Radiographic Examination

History and physical examination should lead the examiner to order x-ray films of the appropriate region. Films will not only confirm the presence or absence of fractures or dislocations in most instances, but will also reveal the type of fracture and the degree of displacement.

Most fractures and dislocations require two x-ray views at 90° angles to each other for proper evaluation; x-rays should usually include the entire length of the bone involved. Some fractures, such as those of the scaphoid and pelvis, require special oblique views to delineate the extent of fracture accurately. Dislocations require two views to determine the true position of the joint components (Fig. 2-3).

When evaluation indicates that fracture is likely in an area known to be difficult to interpret with radiography (*e.g.,* the hip, cervical spine, scaphoid, or immature distal humerus) and the initial x-ray views are normal, the patient should be treated as though the fracture is present.

Fractures and Dislocations 13

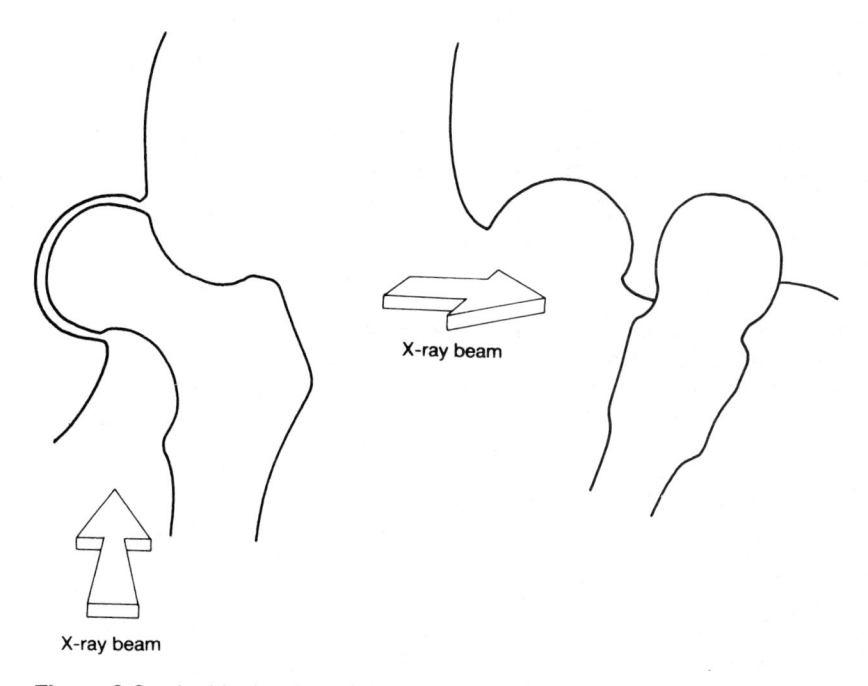

Figure 2-3. In this drawing of x-rays of a dislocated hip, no pathology is apparent in the front view; in the lateral view of the hip dislocation is obvious.

X-ray evaluation repeated in the succeeding 10 to 14 days should verify the presence of fracture by demonstrating either resorption at the fracture line (an early healing phenomenon) or early new-bone formation (callus).

Principles of Fracture Healing

In order to make rational decisions concerning the management of fractures and to understand why certain fractures may exhibit prolonged healing times (delayed union) or, indeed, fail to heal (nonunion), one must understand the basic process of fracture healing.

Bone is a unique tissue. One of its most unusual properties is its capacity to heal by the elaboration of the tissue of which it is composed, bone. Other body tissues heal by the elaboration of fibrous scar; bone heals without scar. This is indeed fortuitous. Most tissues repaired by fibrous scar can function quite well if the damage is not extensive, even though there may be some compromise of tissue strength; bone,

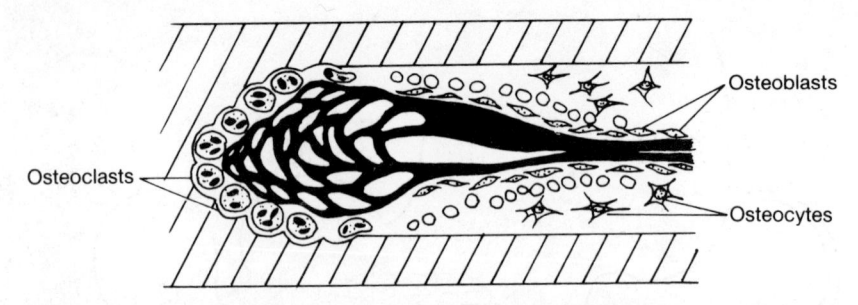

Figure 2-4. This stylized "cutting cone" is moving right to left through bone. At the tip osteoclasts resorb bone; osteoblasts lay down new bone, are engulfed by the matrix they form, and become osteocytes. New osteoblasts are produced from the capillary walls as the cutting cone moves along. (By permission of Smithsonian Institution Press from *Identification of Pathological Conditions in Human Skeletal Remains,* Donald J. Ortner and Walter G. J. Putschar, editors. Smithsonian Contributions to Anthropology Number 28. Figure 17, page 20. Smithsonian Institution, Washington, D.C. Revised edition, 1985)

however, must be restored to normal strength to provide adequate skeletal support and to prevent refracture.

Fracture healing represents a temporary reversion to embryonic bone formation with activation of the membranous and enchondral metaplastic modes and an acceleration of the ongoing mode of cortical bone remodeling. The healing may be divided into two basic types, primary and secondary. These terms are derived from concepts of wound healing in which wounds perfectly approximated heal without interposed granulation tissue (*primary intention*) and wounds with gaps heal with interposed granulation tissue during an early stage (*secondary intention*).

Fractures whose surfaces are closely apposed, well aligned, and rigidly fixed (*e.g.,* with the application of rigid metallic fixation) heal by primary means, that is, by remodeling of bone ends only. The hematoma does not calcify or form bone. The interior cortical bone in adults is remodeled by "cutting cones," capillaries that slowly penetrate the bony substance and create a hole by removing old bone which is then filled with new bone (Fig. 2-4).

Less-rigid fixation (*e.g.,* with a cast) leads to secondary healing; stability around the fracture is, in part, accomplished with an external bridging callus that forms in the hematoma surrounding the fracture. Healing with callus has been shown to produce a stronger early healing, is easier to judge radiographically, and avoids the occasional unpleasant late sequelae associated with insertion of metallic fixation devices.

Secondary fracture healing may be divided into three overlapping phases.

Inflammatory Phase

As in all healing, inflammation plays a role. In bony healing, because of the requirements of structural integrity, the inflammatory response has some unique features. Injury to bone and adjacent soft tissue produces local hemorrhage, which coagulates to form hematoma about the fracture; the usual acute inflammatory response then occurs with vasodilation, edema from plasma exudate, and invasion of acute inflammatory cells (Fig. 2-5). In adults the inflammatory phase lasts for about five days and sets the stage for a proliferative, or reparative, phase.

Proliferative Phase

The hallmark of the proliferative phase is the development of callus, the calcified tissue that forms about a fracture to provide early stabilization (Fig. 2-6). The fracture hematoma is invaded by capillaries along with mesenchymal cells, the connective-tissue progenitor cells. These mesenchymal cells are capable of differentiating into fibroblasts, chondroblasts, and osteoblasts; it is believed that the direction of the differentiation depends upon the nature of the stresses and the condition of the microenvironment. The major source of these mesenchymal cells is the ingrowth of new blood vessels to the fracture site, primarily from surrounding muscle. The mesenchymal cells produce fibrous tissue, cartilage, and immature fiber bone, all of which form the callus tissue.

Bone can develop either directly from fibrous tissue (intramembranous: *e.g.,* periosteal bone formation) or from cartilage (endochondral: *e.g.,* from the epiphyseal plate). Both processes are involved in callus formation. Early in the proliferative phase the periosteum provides an incomplete cover for the hematoma and is a source of osteoblasts, which lay down osteoid on live and necrotic bone fragments. Simultaneously, at the gap of the fracture, where no fragments

16 Trauma

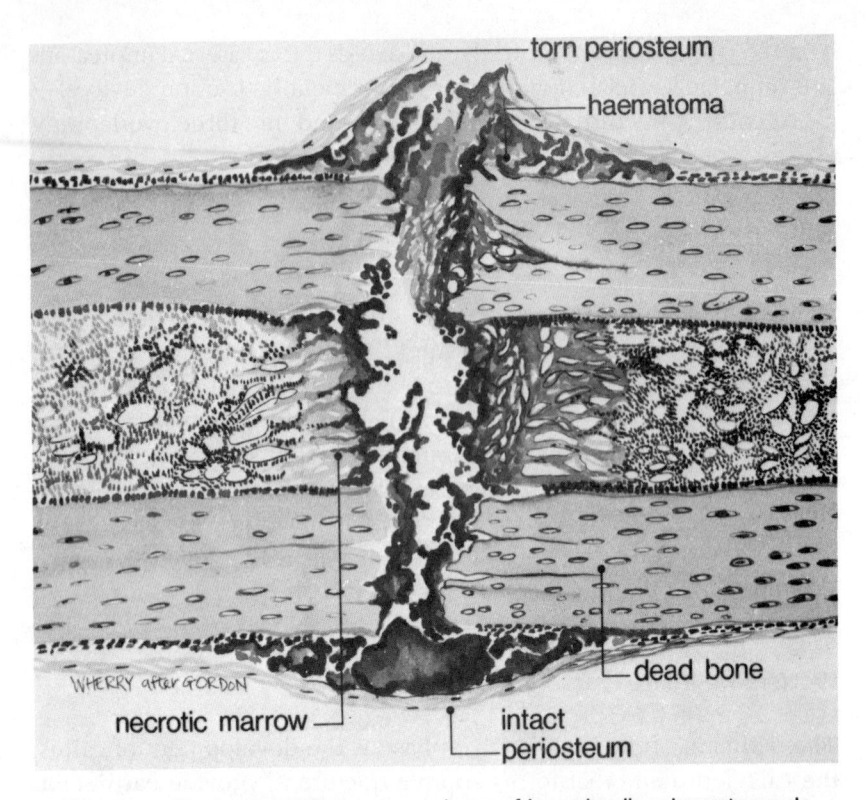

Figure 2-5. During the inflammatory phase of bone healing, hematoma develops around and through broken bone, even when the periosteum remains intact. Hematoma formation is essential for callus formation. (Rockwood CA, Green DP: Fractures in Adults, 2nd ed, p 148. Philadelphia, JB Lippincott, 1984)

exist, the periosteum forms cartilaginous rings around the fragment ends. By approximately the second or third week, this mass will be fairly solid due to a combination of cartilage calcification and periosteal new-bone formation, although some of the cartilage in the callus may remain unchanged. Bone formation proceeds more rapidly in children because their cells are already in a proliferative growing phase. While the external callus is forming, the restoration of medullary blood supply from nutrient and metaphyseal vessels proceeds. As the medullary callus formation is stimulated to further stabilize the fracture, the abundant blood supply of the external callus recedes.

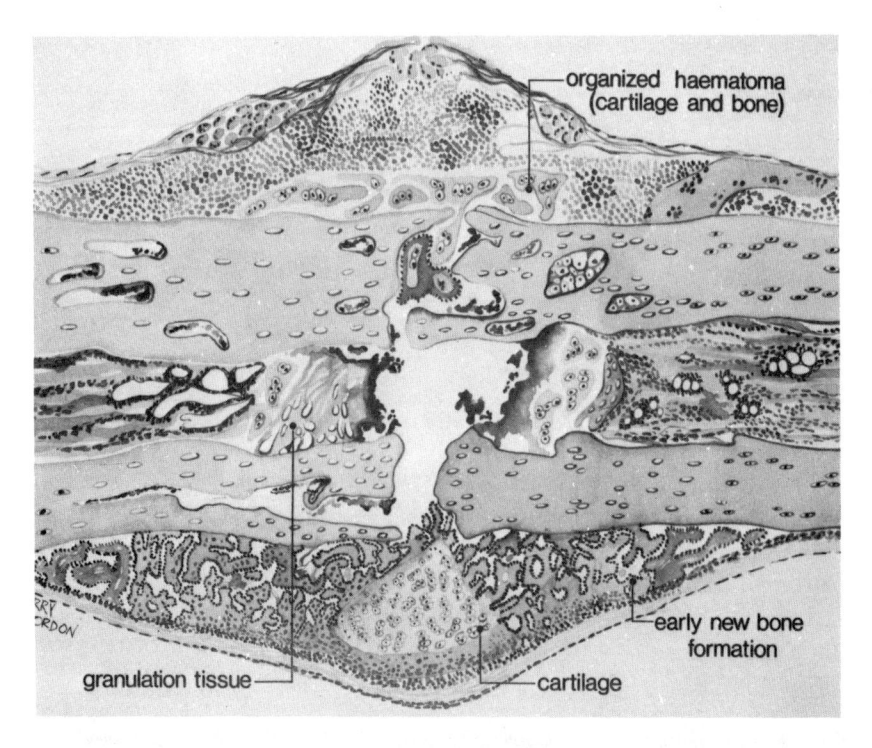

Figure 2-6. In the proliferative phase the hematoma is organized, and by the second or third week will be somewhat "bony" due to cartilage calcification and periosteal new-bone formation. (Rockwood CA, Green DP: Fractures in Adults, 2nd ed, p 149. Philadelphia, JB Lippincott, 1984)

Remodeling Phase

During fracture healing the normal ongoing process of bone remodeling (Fig. 2-7) is greatly accelerated about the fracture and throughout the entire bone. The reconstruction of the bone is accomplished by the gradual resorption of the immobilizing callus by osteoclasts, the deposition of new bone by capillary ingrowth, and osteoblastic bone formation.

Before new bone can replace dead bone (made necrotic by the destruction of its blood supply at the time of fracture), the dead bone must be removed. Thus, remodeling requires osteoclastic activity. As the fracture remodels and the bone returns to its normal strength, the fracture callus is absorbed. The usual sequela of a fracture is complete

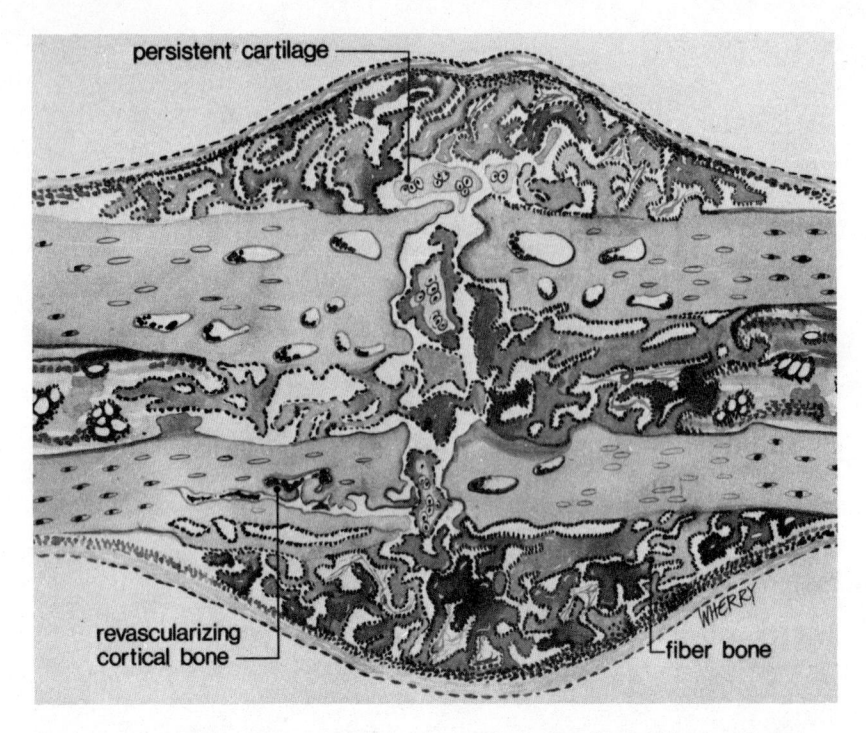

Figure 2-7. During the remodelling phase, the callus is resorbed and new bone is laid by capillary ingrowth and osteoblastic bone formation. (Rockwood CA, Green DP: Fractures in Adults, 2nd ed, p 150. Philadelphia, JB Lippincott, 1984)

or almost-complete restoration of the original structure. This restoration is more complete in the child than in the adult, but several years after a fracture has healed, it is possible, even in an adult, to find no radiographic evidence that it has occurred.

Bone is remodeled along the lines of stress. This process is most dramatic after long-bone fractures in small children, where considerable residual angulation of the fracture may be corrected in a relatively short period of time. Although bone remodeling is active following adult fractures, it does not have the capacity to correct angulatory deformities as in children's fractures.

Cortical bone healing is much slower than cancellous bone healing, where there is a ready source of stem cells from marrow and less bone to resorb. Indeed, well-approximated cancellous bone fractures may be solidly united 4 weeks after a fracture occurs, whereas cortical bone fractures in the adult usually require 8 to 12 weeks or longer to heal. Cancellous bone healing proceeds by the formation of fibrovascular tissue at the fracture site on existing bone trabeculae, whether living or dead, and conversion of this tissue to bone by intramembranous bone formation. This form of healing is really an acceleration of physiological cancellous bone remodeling, an ongoing (but slow) process in normal bone.

Factors Affecting Speed of Healing

A basic requirement for fracture healing is an adequate blood supply since capillary ingrowth provides the source of cells essential for fracture healing. Indeed, the rate of fracture healing depends upon the state of the vascularity in the bone and around the fracture site.

High-velocity injuries, because they impart so much energy, can cause extensive damage not only to the bone but also to the surrounding soft tissues, which are the primary source of blood supply to healing fractures. Thus, nonunion more commonly occurs in severe, high-energy injuries. One should keep in mind the slow healing potential of comminuted fractures, since the fragmentation of bone is usually associated with considerable soft-tissue (and thus vascular) injury.

Significant gaps or interposition of soft tissue (such as muscle) between fracture fragments can mechanically block the formation of bridging callus and can be a cause of nonunion. Fracture fragments must be in relative apposition to heal.

If only one fracture fragment is well vascularized the fracture *can* unite, by a process known as "creeping substitution." Blood supply from the vascularized fragment invades the avascular fragment. Ultimately, necrotic bone is resorbed and living bone deposited. This long and arduous process usually results in union, although delayed. Two common fractures frequently associated with disruption of the blood supply to one fragment are those of the scaphoid and neck of the femur. For this reason these injuries have a high rate of delayed union and nonunion.

It is obvious that capillary ingrowth into the fracture hematoma depends upon holding the healing area relatively quiet. After this initial phase some slight motion at the fracture site stimulates healing. If after a week or two the fracture is braced instead of left in a cast, some motion and early loading of the fracture site occur, and clinically the healing rate is increased. Casts are not "totally immobilizing" and actually allow some compression and bending at the fracture site, since the soft tissues (muscles, fat, etc.) surrounding the bone are somewhat deformable. Compression tends to keep the fragments together, and a certain amount of bending at the fracture site will promote callus formation. Tension at the fracture site, such as that accompanying prolonged excess traction, delays or prevents bony union, as does torsion or shear.

Certain preexisting pathological conditions in bone may also predispose to nonunion. Metastatic malignancy is the most common such pathological entity. It seems likely that extensive destruction of bone by tumor results in the loss of a large part of the osteogenic potential and inhibits revascularization for fracture healing. However, fracture union occurs in some patients despite metastatic malignancy. Radiation necrosis of bone also predisposes to fracture nonunion because the presence of necrotic bone and fibrotic marrow interferes with revascularization.

Infection in fractures is more likely to occur if the skin surrounding the bone is broken. When the skin is broken, the fracture is *open* and requires special treatment. These are usually higher-energy injuries than are *closed* fractures where the skin is not broken. Once the skin is broken, bacteria can contaminate the fracture hematoma as it forms. Of course, the open injury can extend down to the bone, and dirt may actually be embedded in the bone. Nonopen or closed fractures subjected to elective surgical intervention risk the development of postoperative infection. Infection about fractures predisposes to delayed union and nonunion by causing bone and soft-tissue necrosis and retarding the ingrowth of new vascularity in the reparative process.

Principles of Fracture Management

Fractures have a propensity to heal regardless of the type of treatment afforded, even, indeed, in the absence of treatment. The function of the physician in fracture management is to assist the patient in healing the fracture in the shortest time possible and in regaining maximum function of the impaired part. One must be aware of the potential for complications in fracture management and institute preventive measures.

The treatment of fractures may be divided into three phases: emergency management, definitive treatment, and rehabilitation.

Emergency Management

Immediate care of an injured patient involves management of obstructed airway and head and chest injuries, and control of external hemorrhage and shock, before treatment of fractures and dislocations. External hemorrhage is most effectively controlled by applying firm manual pressure to the open wound through a temporary dressing improvised from dressing sponges or the cleanest material available. Local pressure on an extremity wound is more effective and much safer than a tourniquet; a tourniquet applied too tightly or left on too long may sometimes cause tissue necrosis with permanent damage to blood vessels, nerves, and other tissues.

Large volumes of blood may be lost even in closed fractures. Fractures of the femur may be accompanied by the loss of one to two liters of blood, and fractures of the pelvis may result in exsanguination. Any patient who has sustained femoral, pelvic, or multiple fractures should have blood drawn immediately for cross matching. Also, at least one large-bore intravenous catheter should be inserted and kept open should fluid replacement be necessary.

Patients with fractures should be splinted immediately at the site of injury for several reasons: (1) further soft-tissue injury (especially to nerves and vessels) may be averted and closed fractures may be prevented from becoming open by puncture of the skin from within by sharp fracture fragments; (2) immobilization relieves pain by stabilizing the segment and diminishing muscle spasm; (3) splinting may well lower the incidence of fat embolism and shock; and (4) movement and radiographic examination will be more comfortable for the patient.

The slow and steady application of traction is the most effective and least painful way to straighten a grossly deformed extremity. Traction also supports an injured limb while it is being splinted. An injured upper limb is best splinted by being bound to the patient's trunk, and an injured lower limb can be bound to the opposite limb. Temporary limb splints can be improvised from many available objects, including magazines or rolled-up newspapers, umbrellas, and slats of wood padded by any soft material.

Muscle spasm is the body's attempt to immobilize a structure and always occurs with fractures and dislocations. Gentle traction will diminish muscle spasm because the Golgi tendon apparatus, when stimulated with stretching, responds by reflex to inhibit muscle contracture. This protective mechanism, probably designed to prevent rupture of muscles, can be used to stop muscle spasm.

A spinal injury may not be obvious, but can be revealed by the history, symptoms, and testing for local tenderness along the spine and for neurologic signs. The spine should be splinted before the injured patient is moved because movement of an unstable spinal column endangers the spinal cord and nerve roots. Injudicious movement of a patient with an unstable neck or back injury can cause permanent neurologic loss.

Dislocations should be considered emergencies because the stretching of periarticular tissues associated with dislocations can cut off the blood supply to epiphyseal bone, quickly leading to osteonecrosis if the dislocation is not promptly reduced. If muscle spasm can be temporarily dissipated, either with traction or anesthesia, reduction of the joint can usually be accomplished by closed manipulation. If closed manipulation fails or endangers critical structures, such as nerves and arteries, or intra-articular fracture fragments or other structures block reduction, surgical (open) reduction is indicated. After reduction the joint must be kept from redislocating until the periarticular soft tissues that normally maintain joint stability have healed. This generally takes about three weeks.

Definitive Treatment

The definitive treatment of fractures must be delayed until the general condition of the patient has been stabilized. Factors such as age of the patient, site and configuration of the fracture, amount of initial displacement, probable blood supply of the fracture fragments, and functional expectations are important with regard to the choice of therapy.

Certain basic decisions must be made to determine the most appropriate treatment of fractures. Are the present alignment and apposition satisfactory, or does the fracture require a formal reduction to improve the position of the fragments? If so, can the reduction be

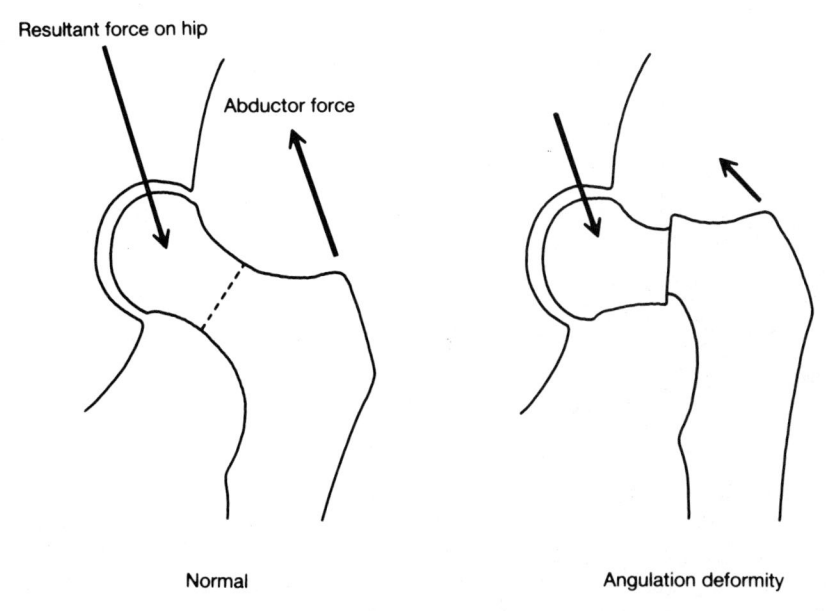

Figure 2-8. A fracture of the femoral neck that heals in varus increases the lever arm through which the abductor muscles function, thereby decreasing the load across the hip joint. (After Radin EL, Simons SR, Rose RM, Paul JL: Practical Biomechanics for the Orthopedic Surgeon, p 124. New York, John Wiley & Sons, 1979)

done closed (manipulatively) or does it require open (surgical) methods? Once adequate reduction is achieved, how can it be maintained until bone healing occurs?

The restoration of maximum musculoskeletal function may, indeed, require the reduction of a fracture. Moreover, reduction can optimize the chance of fracture healing by providing better apposition of fragments; it may also improve the appearance of the injured part. Rotational deformity may cause gait abnormality in the lower extremity and abnormal hand positioning in the upper extremity. Excessive shortening of a leg can produce an abnormal gait. Allowing fractures to heal with excessive angulation may result in impaired muscle function because such angulation changes the effective lever arm through which the muscle works (Fig. 2-8) or may cause abnormal joint loading leading to post-traumatic osteoarthrosis. Intra-articular fractures, fractures that involve the joint, must be accurately reduced to prevent intra-articular stress concentrations, which predispose to late arthrosis.

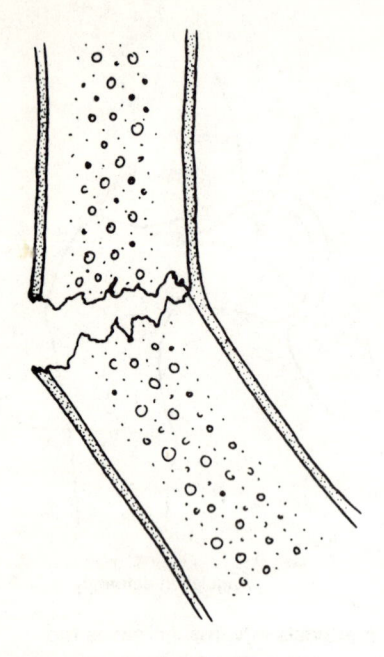

Figure 2-9. Although soft-tissue attachments are usually torn on at least one side of a fracture, they are often intact on the other side.

Fractures can be reduced surgically or by closed methods. The major methods of reduction are discussed below.

Traction. If there is remaining periosteal tissue, or if ligaments or muscle cross the fracture sites, simple traction may reduce the fracture. The soft tissues attached to bone that cross the fracture site contribute to the ability to control the fragments (Fig. 2-9).

Closed Manipulation. If it is possible to gain control of both fracture fragments and obtain adequate muscle relaxation, one can manipulate the fragments into satisfactory position. Sometimes the deforming force must be re-created before the fragments can be levered into a straightened position (Fig. 2-10 A, B).

Manipulation by Surgical Intervention. Direct manipulation of the fracture fragments during surgery is sometimes indicated.

Manipulation Using Skeletal Pins. Percutaneous rigid pins can be drilled into the fracture fragments to aid manipulation. This method is particularly advantageous when it is difficult to obtain control of the fracture fragments easily by other means.

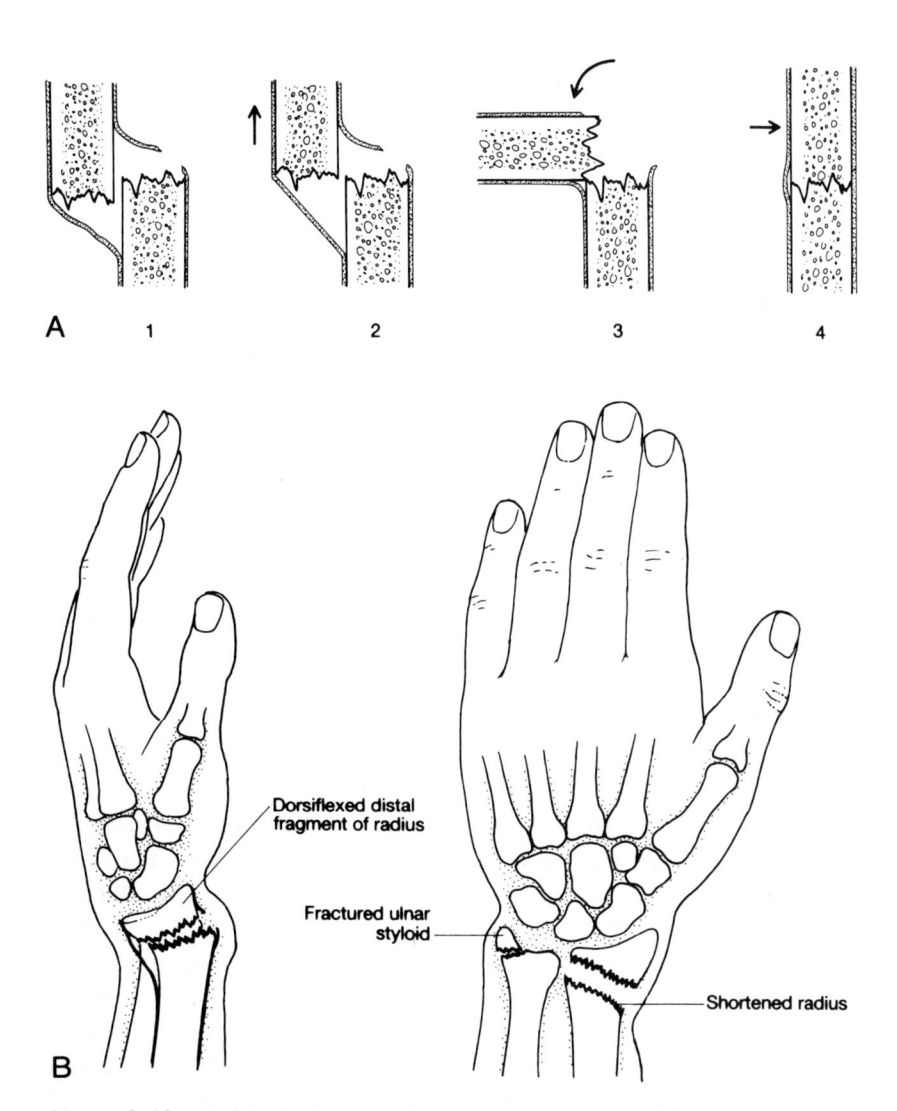

Figure 2-10. *A:* Intact attachments can be used to control fragments during reduction. The fracture is reduced by traction and angulation in order to catch one section of the broken bone on another. The fragments can then be re-aligned. *B:* The most common fracture, a Colles' fracture of the wrist, can usually be reduced by the method outlined in Figure 2-10A.

Methods of Immobilization

Protection. Relatively undisplaced stable fractures in the upper extremity (*e.g.,* impacted fracture of the surgical neck of the humerus) may be treated by a simple sling. In the case of an involved lower extremity, crutches may be used for partial or non-weight bearing.

External Fixation. External fixation of fractures may be achieved by the use of plaster or plastic casts, splints (plaster, metallic, plastic), or fracture braces. Some braces afford relative immobilization of fractures, even though they allow joint motion, because they tightly compress the soft tissues surrounding the fracture.

Continuous Traction. Continuous traction may be applied through the skin by the application of bandages and tape (skin traction) or a metal pin in the bone. This latter form of traction (skeletal traction) is commonly used for comminuted, unstable fractures of the distal femur and humerus.

After an initial period of continuous skeletal traction to produce relative stability, the application of a fracture brace may enable early function.

External Skeletal Fixation. Percutaneous pins are inserted into the bone, usually at some distance from the fracture site. One can manipulate the fragments by manipulating the pins. After adequate reduction has been obtained, a frame can be applied to connect and stabilize the pins. This method affords rigid immobilization of fractures and easy access for wound care. External skeletal fixation is most commonly used for high-energy comminuted fractures with extensive soft-tissue injury necessitating frequent wound care. It is frequently compatible with adjacent joint function and early motion.

Internal Fixation and Open Reduction. This method is usually employed in conjunction with open reduction, which surgically exposes the fracture site, allowing the fragments to be anatomically pieced back together under direct vision. Metallic devices are applied to rigidly secure the fragments and maintain the reduction. A variety of internal fixation devices have been developed, including screws, onlay plates secured to bone by screws (Fig. 2-11), intramedullary nails, pins, and wires.

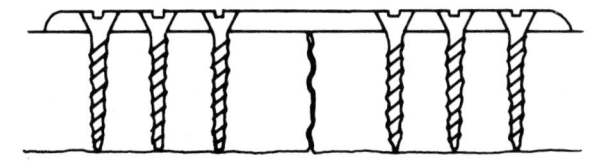

Figure 2-11. Onlay plates secured by screws are one method of internal fixation. (After Radin EL, Simons SR, Rose RM, Paul JL: Practical Biomechanics for the Orthopedic Surgeon, p 73. New York, John Wiley & Sons, 1979)

The major potential advantages of open reduction and internal fixation include the capacity to achieve anatomic reduction of fractures and immediate stability of the fracture. The disadvantages are the attendant risks of anesthesia and infection. In some cases, a second operation is later required to remove the internal fixation device, which, because it is stiffer than the bone, spares the bone from stress. The metal "takes the load" and the bone remains relatively unstressed. Since bone forms in response to stress (Wolff's law) and resorbs when unloaded, protected bone may become osteoporotic and susceptible to refracture.

Open reduction and internal fixation of a fracture are indicated when there is no other way to gain reduction or stability, when anatomic repositioning of articular fragments is necessary in order to minimize subsequent post-traumatic arthrosis after joint fracture, to protect the integrity of an associated arterial or nerve repair, and to allow early function of the patient with a pathological fracture.

Open reduction and internal fixation are commonly carried out for intertrochanteric fractures of the femur, fractures of the tibial plateaus and patella, complex (bi- and tri-malleolar) fractures of the ankle, and shaft fractures of the radius and ulna where control of the fracture fragments is difficult or impossible by other means.

An increasingly popular technique is the use of a closed reduction followed by an intramedullary nailing of certain fractures of long bones that is performed without exposing the fracture site, so that the fracture technically remains "closed" and uncontaminated, reducing the risk of infection. It is performed by reducing the fracture through manipulation and traction, making an incision at some distance from the fracture site, and inserting either a single rigid nail or multiple flexible pins into the medullary cavity across the fracture site to obtain rigid

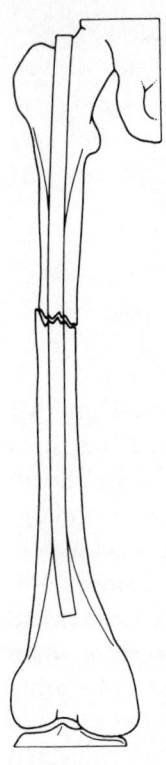

Figure 2-12. Fracture of the shaft of the femur internally fixed with an intramedullary rod. The rod was inserted from the greater trochanter "closed," meaning that the fracture site was not opened. The reduction was carried out at the time of rodding by closed manipulative methods.

fixation. Because this technique involves no surgical disruption of the fracture site, it does not delay the fracture healing as surgical intervention can. Closed intramedullary nailing has been associated with a very high rate of fracture healing and is used commonly for fractures of the midshaft of the femur and tibia (Fig. 2-12).

Multiple injuries, especially those involving several extremities and the chest or the abdomen, have become a major indication for internal fixation, which allows the patient to get out of bed early in convalescence. Such treatment lessens the potentially fatal risks of prolonged bed rest, embolism, and pneumonia.

Open Fractures

As already noted, fractures associated with a break in the skin pose a special problem—the threat of infection—because of potential contamination of the fractured bone and subsequent hematoma. Extensive bone and soft-tissue damage is frequently associated with such open fractures because it usually results from high-energy injuries. Open fractures are, indeed, surgical emergencies! It is crucial that every attempt be made to cleanse the wound as completely and quickly as possible by débridement of the necrotic and contaminated tissue, and lavage to give the bacteria insufficient time to colonize and establish themselves.

When bone is protruding through skin, the first step in emergency treatment should be to cover the exposed bone with saline-soaked, sterile dressings and to immobilize the extremity with appropriate splinting. No attempt should be made to reduce the protruding bone, usually contaminated with foreign material, until the bone can be surgically cleansed; reduction would only seed the wound. These injuries should be reduced in the operating room under sterile conditions.

Fractures in Children

Because of the very active, well-developed periosteum around children's bone and because of the open growth plate at either end of the long bones, the basic principles of caring for injuries in children are somewhat different from those already discussed.

The structure of the growth plate and its position relative to joints make the epiphyseal plate the weakest link in the musculoskeletal system of the child and a common place for fracture. Epiphyseal injuries are usually classified according to the Salter–Harris classification. This classification relates the injury to the adjacent joint and to the growth plate (Fig. 2-13). The exact classification of these injuries, however, is not as important as recognition of the fact that the injuries that occur through the growth plate can create growth disturbance.

Fractures in children are treated by closed reduction, plaster casts, or traction, or by a combination of these methods. Very few of these fractures require open reduction (surgery). The sequelae of fractures in children can be significant, especially if they lead to growth arrest. Growth arrest can be either partial or complete, causing either angular or length deformity. Open reduction is required only for those injuries that involve a joint or the growth plate in such a way that either is displaced. Joint incongruity requires open reduction, just as it does in an adult.

Diaphyseal (bony shaft) injuries in children are also significantly different from similar injuries in adults. A "green stick" fracture is a plastic deformity of the bone that is peculiar to the porous, elastic

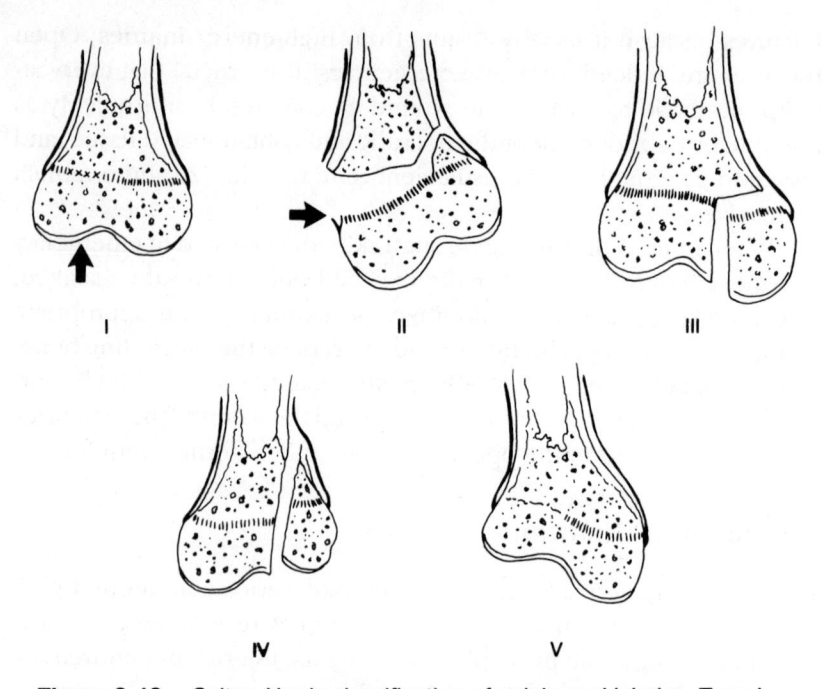

Figure 2-13. Salter–Harris classification of epiphyseal injuries. Type I: minimally displaced; Type II: incomplete separation with a portion of the metaphysis remaining with the epiphysis; Type III: fracture through the epiphysis; Type IV: fracture through the epiphysis and metaphysis; Type V: crush of the epiphyseal plate. (After Salter RB, Horris WR: Injuries involving the epiphyseal plate. J Bone Joint Surg [Am] 45: 587–622, 1963)

bones of children. The bone is bent rather than being broken. Proper treatment requires that the bone be broken completely and then aligned. If this is not done, the bone will angulate further by growing "bent." The sequelae of diaphyseal injuries in children can include overgrowth from overstimulation due to increased blood flow to the injured part. Frequently, bayonet-type apposition of the bone ends is the treatment of choice in fractures prone to such overgrowth. This type of treatment is particularly appropriate for diaphyseal fractures of the femur. Other sequelae of diaphyseal injuries include those related to residual malrotation or angular deformity.

In the forearm of a child, fractures of both bones and fractures of the distal radius are common injuries. Because of the strong, leathery periosteum on the forearm bones, these fractures can almost always be manipulated closed.

Injuries around the elbow pose special problems to children. Supracondylar fractures of the humerus occur in the area immediately above the elbow joint and are troublesome in two ways: (1) there may be significant swelling, which can cause pressure on the nerves and blood vessels in the antecubital space; and (2) there can be significant angular deformity secondary to this injury, causing significant residual malposition of the upper extremity. Fractures around the elbow are the fractures most likely to require surgery in children.

Dislocations

Dislocation of a joint should be considered an urgent problem. Although the condition is not life threatening, the related damage to blood vessels and nerves can be considerable. If the dislocation is not reduced quickly, paralysis or osteonecrosis (death) of the articular end of the bone may follow. In general, x-ray study of the dislocated joint should be carried out before reduction to ensure that there is no associated fracture that may complicate treatment.

The shoulder is the joint most commonly dislocated, probably because it has the least bony stability. The articulation on the scapular side is a disc only 2 inches or so (5 cm) in diameter. The joint is held together by its capsule and associated ligaments. Dislocation of the humeral head from the glenoid most commonly occurs anteriorly and inferiorly and is usually caused by an injury in which the shoulder is forceably abducted and externally rotated. The patient presents with a painful external rotation deformity, usually with the opposite hand supporting the injured arm splinted against the side. Before treatment is considered, it is essential to do a careful neurologic examination. Injury to the axillary nerve and brachial plexus in this situation is quite possible. Also, the dislocation must be differentiated by radiography from a fracture or a fracture–dislocation. Once diagnostic evaluation is complete, gentle manipulative reduction should be performed and repeat radiographic and neurologic exams carried out to be sure the shoulder is properly reduced and that no fracture was caused or neurologic difficulty created by the manipulative maneuver.

Recurrent dislocation of the shoulder is a problem diagnosed frequently in young adults. The younger the patient, the more likely the dislocation is a sign of a congenital weakness of the shoulder joint capsule. When frequent recurrence of shoulder dislocation becomes a functional problem to the patient, surgical reconstruction of the supporting structures is necessary.

The second most common joint to be dislocated is the patellofemoral joint. The patella is prominent on the anterior aspect of the lower extremity and valgus deformity (knock-knees) or recurvatum (back-kneeing) predisposes to this injury. These deformities tend to make the kneecap ride out of its femoral intercondylar groove. Dislocation of the patella may be reduced by the time the patient is brought to the emergency room since the kneecap is subcutaneous and the deformity obvious to the patient. Also, before hemorrhage, swelling, and the associated muscle spasm occur, the patella remains relatively mobile and can be reduced, usually by extending the knee and pushing the patella back. It almost always dislocates to the lateral side. Treatment consists of reduction, if necessary, and immobilization of the leg in a cylinder cast with the knee in extension. In this position, the torn capsule is approximated and will usually heal. Recurrent patellar dislocations suggest incomplete soft-tissue healing or even more usually a bone- or lower-extremity alignment problem that will eventually require surgical correction. Dislocated patellas must be distinguished from rupture of the quadriceps mechanism or patellar tendon, which usually requires surgical repair. The torn ends of these structures will usually not be in continuity when freed because the quadriceps contracts and tends to pull the proximal portion of the rupture up the leg away from its torn mate.

Dislocation of the elbow is an injury common in both children and adults. In adults it is frequently associated with fractures about the elbow. As is true with any dislocation, general anesthesia may be required to obtain sufficient muscle relaxation to effect a gentle manipulative reduction. Once muscle spasm has occurred, a dislocation is usually held rigidly out of place and one of the major tasks of the physician reducing the dislocation is to first diminish the spasm.

Once reduction has been obtained, it is necessary to immobilize the joint in the reduced position until the soft tissues have a chance to heal. This varies from 3 to 6 weeks depending on the joint.

Rehabilitation

As soon as a fracture has been reduced and immobilized, rehabilitation should begin. The patient must be warned about the dangers that may accompany fracture treatment, especially increased swelling and loss of sensation resulting from too-tight casts and bandages. The patient should also be instructed in an appropriate exercise program in order to maintain joint and muscle function in the involved extremity during the period of immobilization. Lack of motion in the presence of edema and hematoma can lead to permanent scarring and loss of function. For example, impacted fractures of the surgical neck of the humerus invariably heal, but restricted shoulder motion associated with 4 to 6 weeks in a sling can leave the patient with a stiff shoulder and a lifelong functional limitation. Institution of shoulder exercises as soon as possible after the immobilization has begun can obviate this serious complication.

After dislocations, full, unrestricted motion cannot commence until the soft tissues torn by the injury have healed; otherwise recurrent dislocation may occur. When immobilizing devices applied for either the treatment of fractures or dislocations are removed, a more extensive exercise program is prescribed. It is important to recognize the great variation of human response to the rehabilitation process. Temporary disability has a socioeconomic impact on a patient, and the physician must be aware of this and prepared to deal with it.

Chapter 3

Injuries of the Hand

David A. Labosky

The human hand is a unique and complex biomechanical instrument possessing a vast spectrum of functional abilities. The hand is capable of activities ranging from simple grasp to concert piano playing. Endowed with such versatility, the hand lends itself to a wide variety of potentially dangerous tasks, and hand injuries are common. In fact, the hand is injured more frequently than any other part of the body, and since the hand is a basic unit of human productivity, loss of its function is a serious disability.

The physician's primary goal in the treatment of hand injuries should be preservation of hand function. The final outcome of treatment frequently depends on the quality of care during the first few hours, a time when crucial decisions must be made. Thus, it behooves every medical student, especially those planning careers in primary care, to acquire a basic understanding of the principles of the treatment of hand injuries.

The basis for treatment of hand problems is, of course, knowledge of the hand's anatomy. Excellent texts are available as reference sources. In this synopsis we will try to teach this anatomy as it relates to common clinical problems. We will also attempt to present an organized, systematic approach to evaluating hand problems.

Evaluation of Hand Injury

As with fractures and dislocations, a medical history must be taken and a physical examination carried out in order to evaluate a hand injury. All potentially injured structures should be examined to avoid overlooking or misdiagnosing even a seemingly trivial problem. Delay in the treatment of injuries such as tendon lacerations can have serious effects on hand function.

History

The medical history of an injured hand should attempt to answer three questions—How? When? and Where?

The patient's description of how the hand injury occurred will usually include the nature of the injuring force. This will provide some insight into possible tissue trauma. Crush or burn injury usually involves small-vessel damage resulting in tissue necrosis beyond obvious margins. Glass lacerations can present with rather innocuous looking wounds that may conceal extensive damage to underlying structures. Penetrating injuries frequently result in damage to deep structures remote from the skin wound.

The span of time between the injury and the start of treatment should be carefully documented since damage can progress. For example, wound contamination can cause infection if treatment is delayed beyond 6 hours. Edema in the hand increases the tendency for joints to adopt positions that predispose to late contracture. Blood vessel damage accompanying displaced fractures or lacerations can result in irreversible changes. A part rendered ischemic by vascular damage or amputation becomes unsalvageable after a period of time.

Documentation of where an injury took place can be significant in a number of ways. If the injury occurred on the job, the patient may be entitled to compensation. Injuries occurring in dirty environments (farms, butcher shops, poultry-processing plants, the side of the road, etc.) have a greater potential for infection.

Examination

Observation of the normal resting attitude of the hand can provide a great deal of information. With the wrist in relaxed dorsiflexion, the fingers fall passively into moderate flexion (Fig. 3-1). When the wrist is allowed to fall passively into flexion, the fingers extend (Fig. 3-2). This is secondary to the resting tension in the myotendinous units that control finger extension and flexion. If one of the tendons is cut, the affected finger loses its normal resting attitude (Fig. 3-3).

Consider all anatomic structures that lie beneath the injury; these,

Injuries of the Hand   37

Figure 3-1. With the wrist in relaxed dorsiflexion, the fingers fall passively into moderate flexion.

Figure 3-2. When the wrist is allowed to fall passively into flexion, the fingers extend.

too, may be damaged. Lacerations frequently transect tendons, nerves, and arteries. Crush injuries fracture bones, disrupt joints, and devitalize soft tissues.

Inspection is also an important part of the initial evaluation, but the physician should resist the temptation to first look into the wound to see if tendons and nerves are lacerated. More information can be acquired through the careful and systematic examination of all structures distal to the injury. Once a sterile dressing has been applied,

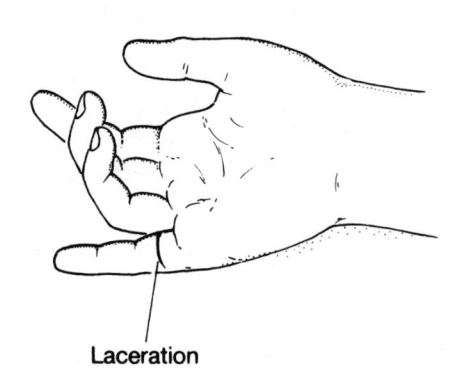

Figure 3-3. If one of the tendons is cut, the affected finger loses its normal resting attitude.

Laceration

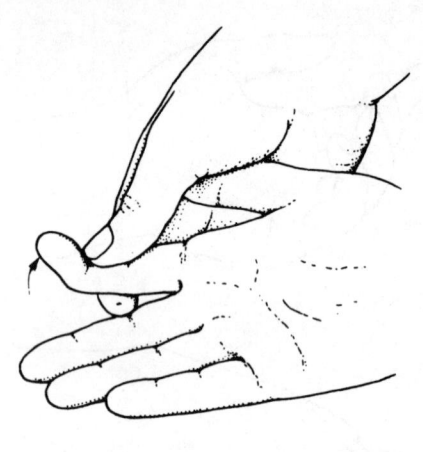

Figure 3-4. Flexor digitorum profundus function is tested by immobilizing all the phalanges proximal to the distal interphalangeal joint and asking the patient to actively flex that joint.

bleeding can usually be controlled by direct pressure. No attempt should be made to clamp "bleeders" in the emergency room; it is all too easy to inadvertently crush a previously uninjured structure. Again, test all anatomic structures distal to the injury, including tendon, nerve, vessel, as well as joint function. Each of the four fingers has two flexor tendons: flexor digitorum profundus and flexor digitorum superficialis. The thumb has only one extrinsic flexor tendon: flexor pollicis longus. To test flexor digitorum profundus function, immobilize all joints proximal to the *distal interphalangeal joint* (DIP) and ask the patient to actively flex that joint (Fig. 3-4). If the tendon is cut, the patient will not be able to flex the end of the finger. Test flexor digitorum superficialis function by holding all fingers except the one under examination in full extension and asking the patient to flex that finger (Fig. 3-5). An intact flexor digitorum superficialis tendon will flex only

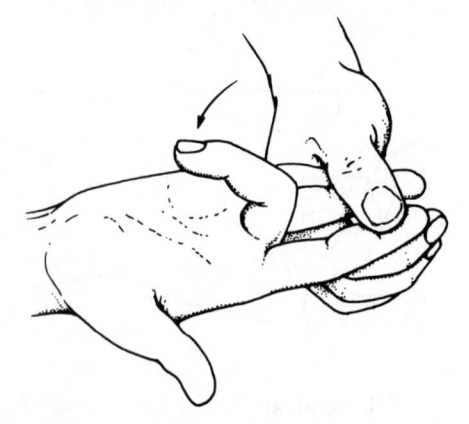

Figure 3-5. Flexor digitorum superficialis function is tested by holding all the fingers but one in extension and asking the patient to flex that finger.

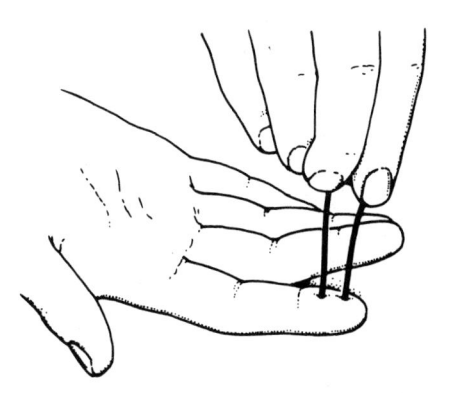

Figure 3-6. Two-point discrimination can be tested with a paper clip.

the *proximal interphalangeal joint* (PIP). To test common digital extensor tendon function, hold the wrist in neutral position and ask the patient to extend the *metacarpophalangeal* (MCP) *joint.* If the tendon is cut, the patient will be unable to fully extend the finger. Test motor control of each joint distal to the injury sequentially.

Test nerve function distal to injury by sensation and muscle activity. Testing light touch with a whisp of cotton is much more effective than pin-prick evaluation. Two-point discrimination tested with a bent paper clip can provide quantitative evaluation of sensation. The paper clip should be bent so that the two ends contact the fingertip at the same time (Fig. 3-6). The patient is asked to distinguish one point of touch from two when the examiner presses the paper clip tips to the finger pulp just hard enough to blanch the skin. The opposite, normal hand can be used as a control in adjusting the ends of the paper clip apart or together to establish the threshold of the patient's ability to discriminate between one and two points touching the skin.

The *median nerve* supplies the thumb and the index and long fingers, as well as half of the ring finger (Fig. 3-7). The autonomous zone for the median nerve is the radial side of index-finger pulp. A nerve's autonomous zone is the area of skin that will always be innervated by that nerve despite variations caused by anatomic anomalies. The *ulnar nerve* supplies half the ring finger and the small finger (autonomous zone: ulnar side of small-finger pulp). The *radial nerve* supplies the dorsum of the hand (autonomous zone: dorsal first web space between thumb and index finger).

Test the motor function of all neuromuscular units distal to the injury. For the median nerve, test the abductor pollicis brevis (palmar abduction of thumb). For the ulnar nerve, test the interossei (ability

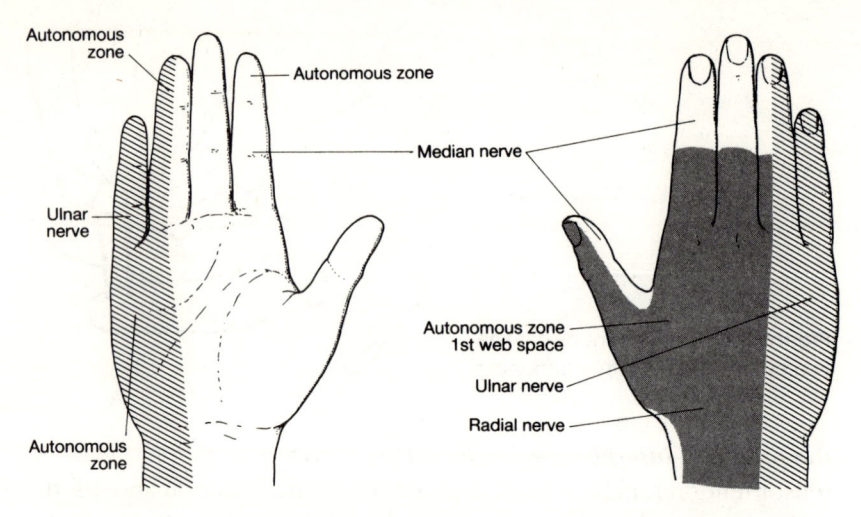

Figure 3-7. Sensory territories of the median (unshaded), ulnar (crosshatched), and radial (dark-colored) nerves.

to spread and bring together fingers, ability to pinch thumb to index finger with force). For the radial nerve, test the extension and abduction of the thumb.

Evaluate the vascular supply to the hand by color of fingers, capillary refill time (blanch and refill of nail bed or finger pulp), and palpation of radial and ulnar arteries.

Types of Hand Injuries

Flexor Tendon Injuries

Since the functional result after repair of flexor tendons differs greatly depending upon the area on the hand or wrist where the lacerations occurred, the hand has been divided into zones for purposes of classifying tendon lacerations (Fig. 3-8). The region between the DIP flexion crease and distalpalmar crease has been designated "no man's land" because of the very dense fibro-osseous tunnel through which the tendons pass in this area. The fibro-osseous tunnel contains a set of pullies that guide the tendon around the concave side of the finger as it flexes (Fig. 3-9). During healing of a tendon laceration in this area, the tendon repair site easily becomes attached by fibrous scar to tunnel walls. This tethers the tendon to the rigidly fixed tendon sheath,

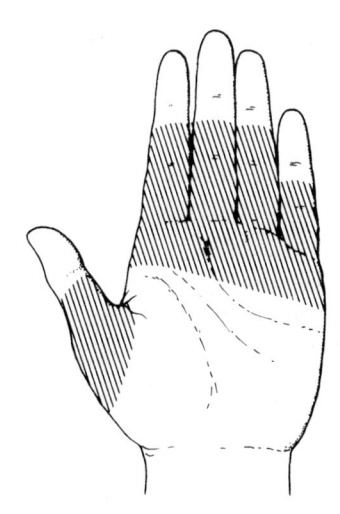

Figure 3-8. Cross-hatched area is "no man's land," where flexor tendon laceration repairs are prone to scar down.

restricting gliding of the tendon and thus preventing full flexion and extension of the finger. Many techniques are used to minimize this scarring and subsequent loss of function. With injuries involving these tendons, meticulous attention to detail and accurate tendon approximation at surgery are particularly important to ultimate function. Because of the serious functional consequences of flexor tendon injuries and the technical difficulties associated with effective repair, tendon laceration should be treated early by qualified surgeons in the controlled environment of the operating room.

The level of recovery of function following flexor tendon repair depends not only upon the surgeon's skill but also upon the rehabilitation program instituted after surgery. A careful plan of splinting and passive and active exercises minimizes restriction of tendon excursion by scarring and joint contracture. This program of therapy takes into consideration the healing process occurring within the tendon and

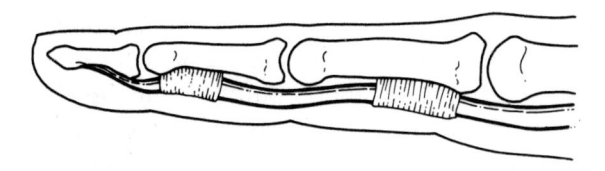

Figure 3-9. Pulley system of the digital flexor tendon sheath.

wound. The functional recovery of a patient with a flexor tendon laceration is as dependent on the attention of a therapist trained in the care of hand rehabilitation as it is on the training and expertise of the surgeon.

Extensor Tendon Injuries

Extensor tendons on the dorsum of the hand are surrounded by loose connective tissue with no restrictive tendon sheath. Thus, as a rule, simple laceration of these structures is easier to treat than injuries to flexor tendons and can be handled by direct surgical repair. A laceration over the MCP joint or on the dorsum of the hand can transect a common digital extensor tendon, resulting in loss of ability to extend the MCP joint. The PIP and DIP joints, however, will continue to extend by action of the intrinsic muscles through lateral bands and terminal tendon (Fig. 3-10). The dorsal surface of the hand and those of the fingers are very much subject to blunt trauma. Because of this, a variety of unique injuries are associated with the extensor tendons.

Human Bite Injury (Clenched-Fist Injury). Beware of a ragged laceration over the knuckles. The blow of a clenched fist to the mouth frequently results in laceration of the patient's hand on the other person's teeth. Because of the virulent organisms present in human saliva, chance of serious infection is high if such a wound is mishandled. All of these wounds must be examined radiographically to evaluate for fracture or retention of a piece of tooth in the wound. Surgical exploration is mandatory to evaluate depth of wound and potential joint and tendon involvement. Appropriate surgical treatment of injured structures is then performed; wounds are not sutured closed. Antibiotics should be given. The most common infecting organism is *Staphylococcus aureus.*

Boutonniere Deformity. This deformity consists of a flexion contracture of the PIP joint and an extension contracture of the DIP joint (Fig. 3-11). It is a result of either laceration or blunt disruption of the common extensor tendon at its insertion on the base of a middle phalanx. The attendant imbalance of tendon pull crossing the PIP joint is the source of the deformity. Early treatment of the tendon disruption can prevent development of the deformity. Lacerated tendon should be surgically repaired and splinted for 5 weeks with the PIP in exten-

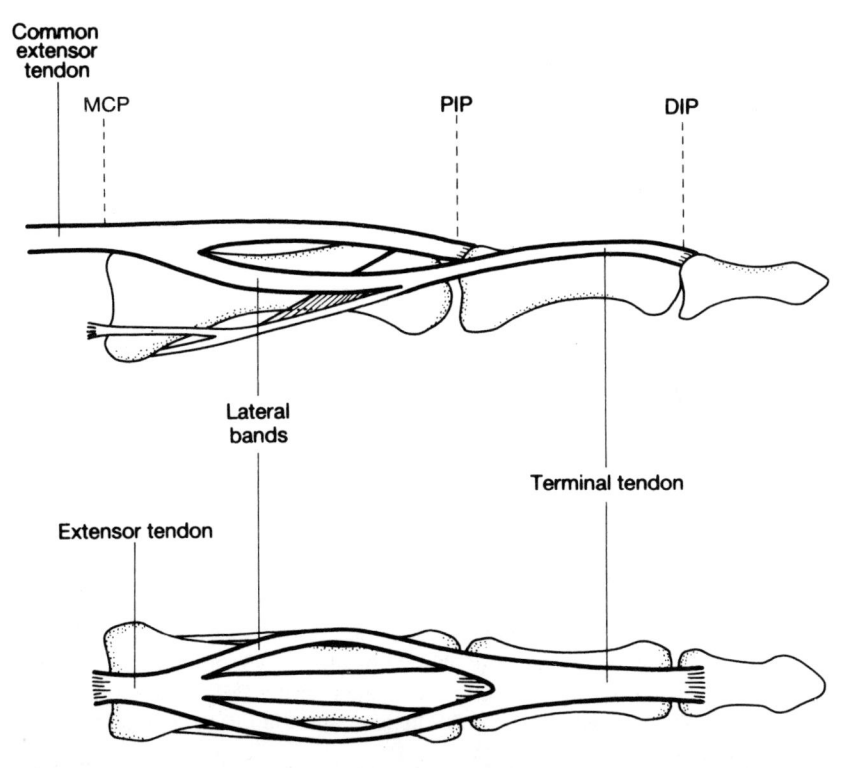

Figure 3-10. The extensor mechanism of the finger includes the common extensor tendon and lateral bands joined by the retinacular fibers of the extensor mechanism. The PIP is extended by the common extensor and lateral band, and the DIP is extended by the conjoined slips of the lateral bands which form a terminal tendon.

sion. Blunt injury can be treated with simple extension splinting for 5 to 7 weeks.

Mallet Deformity (Dropped Finger, Baseball Finger). Mallet finger is usually the result of a forceful passive flexion of the DIP or a blow on the end of the finger. It frequently occurs when a baseball or basketball is caught on the end of the finger. It can also occur secondary to a sharp laceration or crushing injury at the DIP joint (Fig. 3-12A). The injury either disrupts the terminal extensor tendon that inserts at the base of the distal phalanx, or it fractures the distal phalanx at the insertion of the tendon or through the joint surface. This results in loss

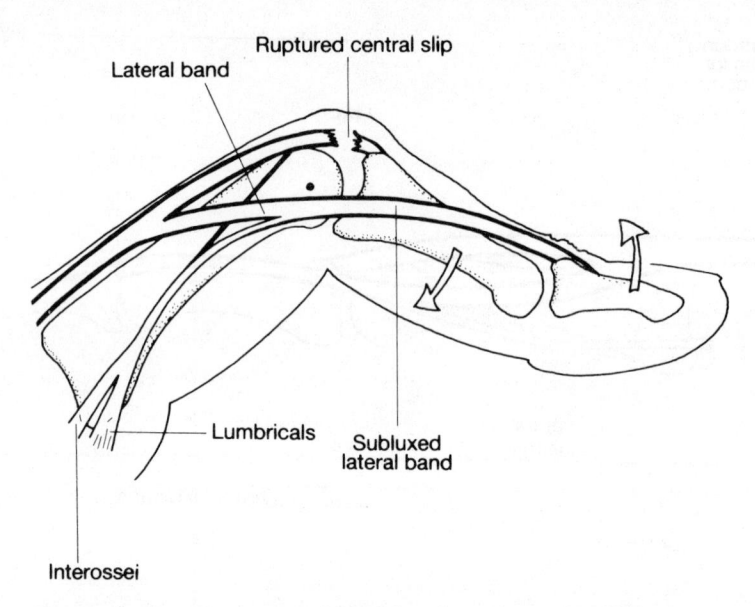

Figure 3-11. The boutonniere deformity occurs when the common extensor insertion ruptures, and the dorsal fibers of the extensor mechanism are no longer able to maintain the lateral bands in the position dorsal to the center of rotation of the PIP. The lateral bands slip volar and become PIP flexors, and the PIP cannot be actively extended.

of extensor force. The flexor tendons then pull the DIP joint into flexion. Treatment of the closed injury is to splint the DIP joint (Fig. 3-12B) in full extension for 6 to 8 weeks. Care must be taken to avoid pressure damage to the skin on the dorsum of the DIP joint secondary to the splinting process. Since the mallet injury can involve significant fracture of the articular surface of the distal phalanx, an x-ray view of the DIP joint should be obtained.

Crush Injuries and Lacerations. Crush injuries with phalangeal fractures and disruption of extensor mechanism over the PIP joint are a common occurrence, particularly in industrial accidents. When a disrupted extensor mechanism heals along with a fracture, the tendons tend to adhere to one another, resulting in restriction of motion. This type of injury presents a difficult therapeutic and surgical problem.

On the dorsum of the wrist the nine extrinsic extensor tendons and three wrist extensors pass through six fibro-osseous compartments similar to the flexor tendon sheaths (Fig. 3-13). Lacerations in this area

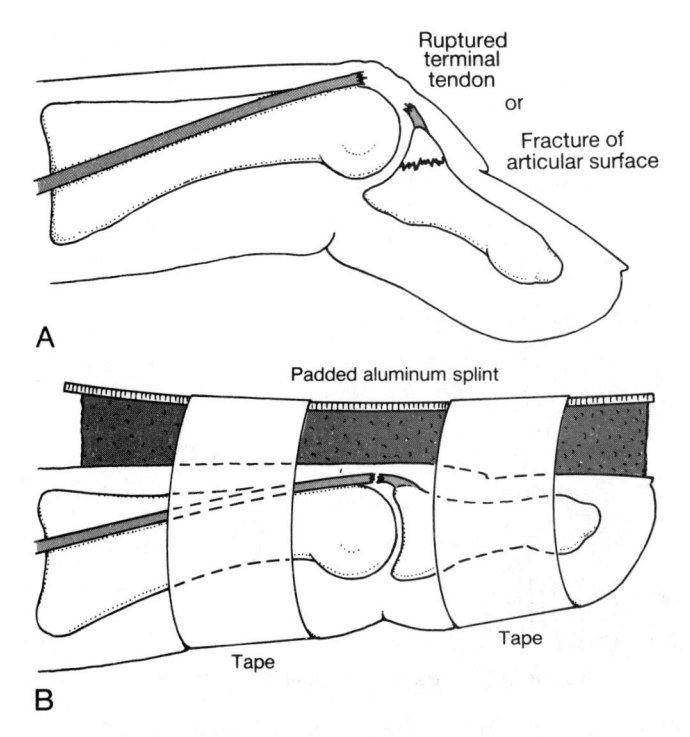

Figure 3-12. *A:* The mallet deformity occurs when the terminal tendon either ruptures or avulses its insertion. Active extension to the DIP is lost, and the joint droops into flexion from the pull of the normal flexor tendons. *B:* DIP joints splinted in extension for mallet deformity.

of the wrist are uncommon and thus present fewer scarring and loss-of-excursion problems than lacerations on the flexor side of the hand. Most extensor tendon lacerations occur on the dorsum of the hand, where surrounding tissues are loose and adhesion is uncommon.

De Quervain's Tenosynovitis. This is a nonspecific tenosynovitis involving the extensor pollicis brevis and abductor pollicis longus tendons in the first dorsal (extensor tendon) compartment. The patient complains of pain and tenderness in the area of the radial styloid (location of the first dorsal compartment). Pain is aggravated by forceful thumb radial abduction (abduction of the thumb away from the radial side of the radius) and dorsiflexion of the wrist. The Finkelstein test, performed by asking the patient to grasp his thumb into his palm and

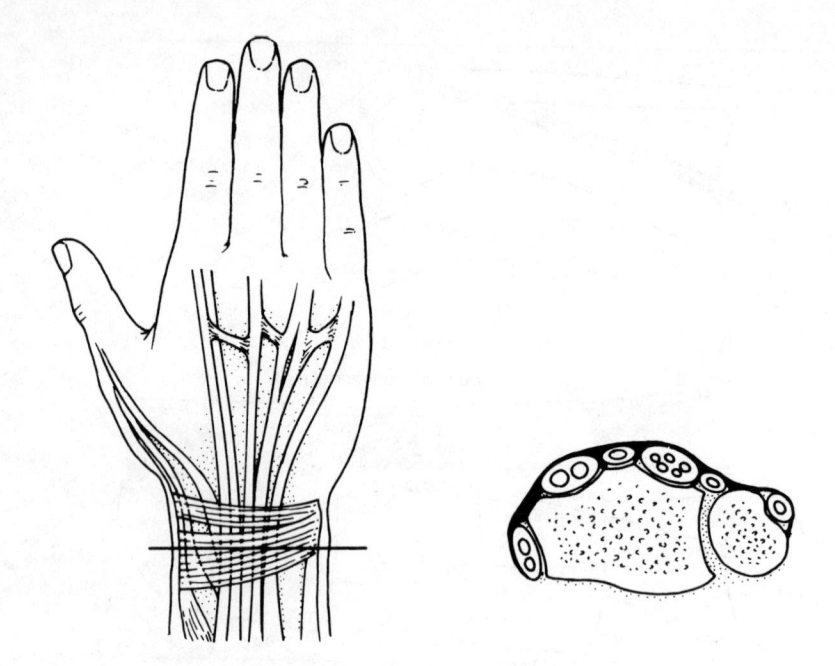

Figure 3-13. Extensor retinaculum of the wrist.

passively deviating the wrist in an ulnar direction, produces pain in the area of the radial styloid (Fig. 3-14).

Treatment consists of splint immobilization and oral anti-inflammatory medication for mild cases. More severe cases will usually respond to steroid injection in the first dorsal compartment; if this fails, the compartment can be released surgically.

It is important to distinguish De Quervain's tenosynovitis from the common arthrosis of the trapeziometacarpal or basal joint of the thumb. With either condition, the patient experiences pain at the base of the thumb. Pain associated with manipulation of the basal joint suggests a diagnosis of arthrosis. This can be confirmed by an x-ray view of the joint.

Trigger Finger (and Trigger Thumb). This is a condition similar in pathophysiology to De Quervain's tenosynovitis. Tenosynovitis involving the flexor tendons at the level of the first pulley (at the MCP joint level) produces a localized swelling of the tendon that becomes caught or stuck as it passes through the narrow pulley in flexion and extension. The finger may snap or trigger into extension because the

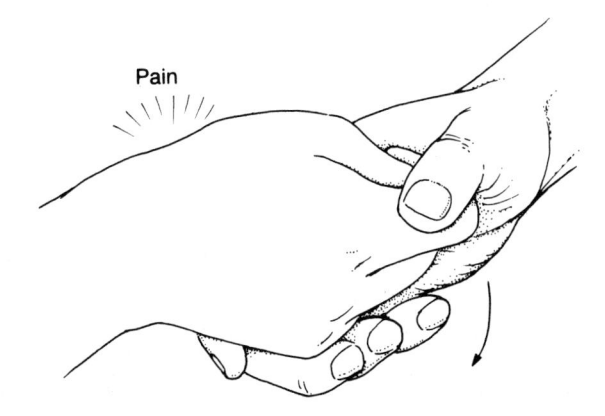

Figure 3-14. Finkelstein test for De Quervain's tenosynovitis.

relatively weaker extensor muscles have difficulty pulling the tendon nodule through the pulley; sometimes the patient must passively pull the finger into extension. Pressure over the flexor tendon at the MCP joint causes pain.

Treatment consists of steroid injection into the tendon sheath or, if injection fails, surgical release of the first pulley.

Nerve Injuries

Each of the three nerves of the hand contains both motor and sensory fascicles and, therefore, injury can involve both components. Nerve lacerations are devastating injuries that require months to heal, even with prompt, appropriate treatment.

The three degrees of nerve injury include neurapraxia, axonotmesis, and neurotmesis. *Neurapraxia* is a first-degree injury in which there is loss of conduction in the axion but not loss of continuity. Simply put, it is a bruise or contusion of the nerve. Recovery is usually complete, occurring within three months. *Axonotmesis* is a second-degree injury in which the axons are damaged and wallerian degeneration occurs. Recovery in this type of injury can be complete, but it takes a great deal of time for axons to regenerate from the site of injury to the end organ innervated. *Neurotmesis* is a complete disruption of the nerve, including axons and neural sheath. An example is a laceration of a nerve. This type of injury requires surgical repair. After the repair,

48 Trauma

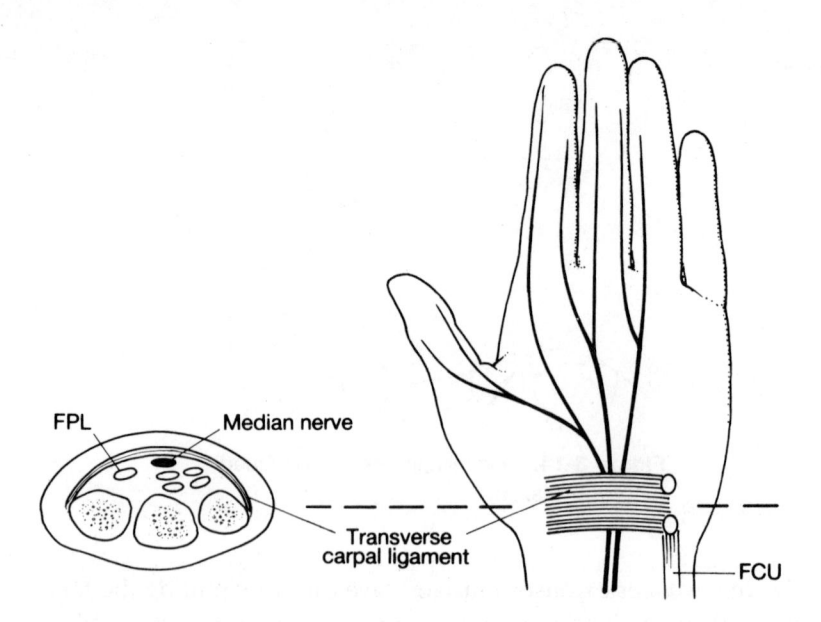

Figure 3-15. The carpal canal contains the nine extrinsic flexor tendons (FPL, four FDSs, four FDPs) and the median nerve. This rigid compartment is bounded by the transverse carpal ligament as its roof, the hook of hamate and tubercle of the scaphoid as its walls, and the carpal bones as its floor.

regeneration of the nerve occurs, progressing very slowly from the site of repair to the end organ.

Carpal Tunnel Syndrome. This is the most common example of a compression neuropathy. The median nerve resides in the unyielding carpal canal with all the flexor tendons of the fingers (Fig. 3-15). Any process that decreases volume in this narrow canal or increases the size of its contents can precipitate carpal tunnel syndrome by causing pressure on the median nerve. These processes include inflammatory and degenerative conditions such as nonspecific tenosynovitis, rheumatoid tenosynovitis, gout, and amyloidosis; post-traumatic conditions such as those following Colles' fracture, wrist dislocation, and capitate fracture; and systemic conditions such as hypothyroidism, acromegaly, obesity, pregnancy, and diabetes.

The typical case of carpal tunnel syndrome often presents with such a classic series of symptoms that diagnosis can be established on the basis of the history. A majority of the patients are females past 40 years of age. Initial symptoms are tingling and numbness in the median innervated fingers. Frequently the patient is awakened from sleep with pain and numbness in the hand. The symptoms are usually relieved by shaking or manipulating the hand. Pain may involve the hand and wrist, and may radiate up the forearm into the arm and shoulder.

The physical examination for carpal tunnel syndrome often reveals tenderness when pressure is applied directly over the carpal canal. *Tinel's sign,* paresthesia (usually tingling) in the median distribution, is elicited by tapping over the inflamed, compressed segment of the median nerve. A positive wrist-flexion test (*Phalen's test*) is elicited when the patient's symptoms are precipitated by maintenance of the wrist in acute volar flexion for 60 seconds or less. Sensory changes in the median nerve distribution (light touch, two-point discrimination) can sometimes be elicited. If the damage to the nerve has progressed sufficiently, atrophy and weakness of the median innervated thenar muscles can be found. These muscles are the opponens pollicis, abductor pollicis brevis, and one half of the flexor pollicis brevis. Testing of median intrinsic function is best done by asking the patient to abduct his thumb away from the palm. This tests the abductor pollicis brevis. Electromyographic changes indicative of carpal tunnel syndrome include a decrease in sensory and motor conduction velocities of the median nerve across the wrist and signs of denervation in the abductor pollicis brevis.

In early cases some relief can be obtained by splinting the wrist in the functional position or by restricting activity. Steroid injection in the carpal canal can decrease swelling, which will relieve symptoms temporarily. In pregnancy, symptoms almost always abate after delivery. If there is evidence of marked sensory change, marked decrease in nerve conduction velocity, or muscle atrophy, or if conservative measures fail, surgical release of the transverse carpal ligament is indicated. This allows the median nerve more room in the carpal canal, preventing recurrent compression.

Cubital Tunnel Syndrome. This occurs when the ulnar nerve becomes inflamed as it passes the medial epicondyle of the elbow. In this situation the nerve is not entrapped in an unyielding canal (as in the carpal tunnel syndrome). Rather, it is subjected to repetitive trauma because its very superficial location, tethered over the bony prominence at a very mobile joint, predisposes it to inflammation and fibrosis.

Treatment, as with other inflammatory processes, begins with rest,

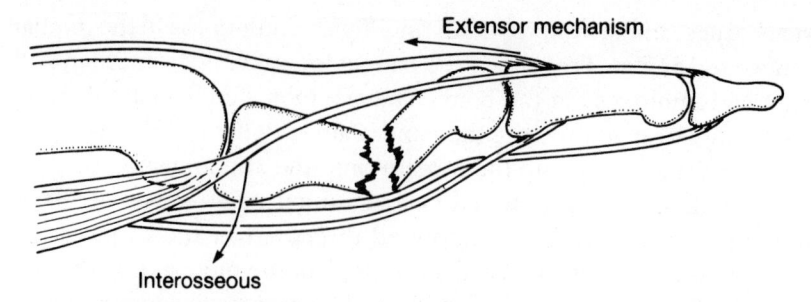

Figure 3-16. The proximal phalanx fracture tends to angulate with the apex of angulation volar because the interosseous muscle flexes the proximal fragment and the pull of the extensors extends the distal fragment.

immobilization, and anti-inflammatory medication. If this fails or if the patient develops weakness or atrophy of the ulnar innervated intrinsic muscles, surgical release of the nerve becomes necessary.

Common Fractures and Dislocations

Fractures involving the hand are frequently obvious by virtue of gross deformity. With any significant trauma to the hand or wrist, radiographic examination is an essential part of the diagnostic workup. X-ray views must include at least a proper posterior–anterior and a true lateral view of the affected part. There is no reason to x-ray the entire hand if the injury involves only a finger. If the whole hand is x-rayed, one is more likely to get a poor lateral view of the injured finger.

Once diagnosis is established, the next step should be to obtain and maintain adequate reduction of the fracture. To do this the physician must consider the fact that the deformity is a result not only of the original injuring mechanism but also of forces of the musculotendinous structures acting across the fracture site (Fig. 3-16). Reduction must control rotation as well as angulation at the fracture site. To determine rotation, flex the MCP joints with the PIP and DIP joints extended and check that the fingernails line up (Fig. 3-17*A*). When the PIP and DIP joints are flexed as well, all the fingers should point toward the tubercle of the scaphoid (Fig. 3-17*B*). Once reduction is obtained, instability or muscle forces acting to deform the fracture may necessitate internal fixation. In most cases, however, external splinting with a partial or a full cast is sufficient to maintain reduction. The external

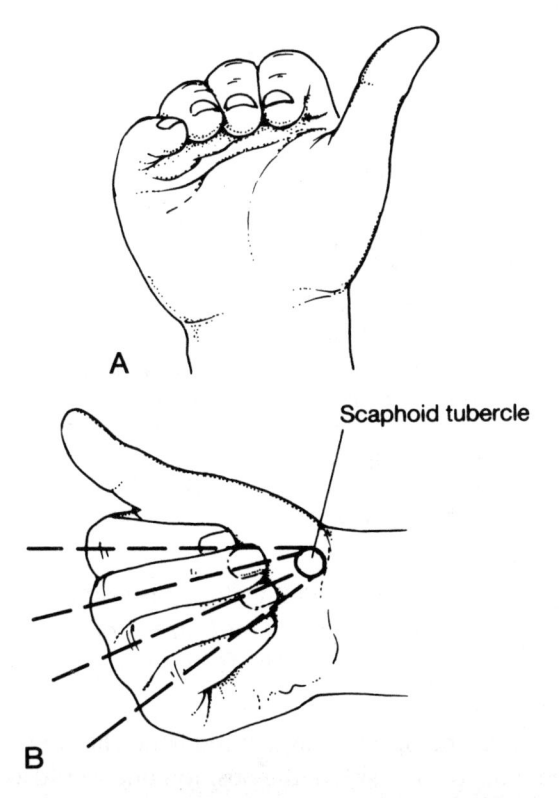

Figure 3-17. *A:* With the MCPs flexed and the PIPs and DIPs straight, all the fingernails line up. If a phalanx fracture is rotated, the nail of the rotated finger will not align with the rest. *B:* With the MCPs and PIPs and DIPs flexed, all the fingers point in the direction of the tubercles of the scaphoid. A rotated metacarpal fracture would disrupt alignment of the affected finger.

support must be maintained until the fracture has healed sufficiently to provide stability and allow early guarded joint motion of the affected fingers and hand. Since the first concern in treatment of hand injuries is the preservation of function, joint mobilization should be a high priority when dealing with hand fractures.

The following rules should be followed:

1. Immobilize only those fingers and joints necessary to maintain reduction.

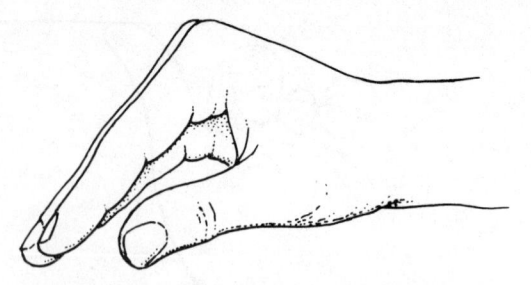

Figure 3-18. Intrinsic-plus position is the position adopted by the hand when the interossei and lumbricals are contracting. The MCPs are flexed and the PIPs and DIPs are extended. Here the ligaments of these joints are in their longest state and are less likely to be contracted if the hand is immobilized in this position for a long period of time.

2. When possible, immobilize joints in a position in which ligaments and capsules are in their longest, or stretched, state.
3. Mobilize the joints as soon as the fracture is stable enough to allow it.

Rule 2 contradicts the old dictum that the hand should be splinted in the so-called functional position, the position one would assume when holding a baseball. While this may be functional for holding baseballs, the MCP joints are in extension, allowing the lax collateral ligaments to become contracted, and the PIP and DIP joints are in flexion, predisposing them to contracture as well. The more appropriate position is called the *position of functional rehabilitation,* with the MCP joints flexed 70° and the PIP and DIP joints flexed only 10 to 15° (Fig. 3-18). This position maintains the collateral ligaments at their lengthened state to allow early joint rehabilitation.

Proximal Phalanx Fracture. This type of fracture frequently presents a problem because of angulation (see Fig. 3-16). The interosseous muscles pull the proximal fracture fragment in flexion, and the common extensor tendon and lateral bands pull the distal fragment into extension. Pin fixation is often necessary.

PIP Joint Fracture Dislocation. This frequently misdiagnosed injury has come to be called "coach's finger." The classic history tells of a football player who emerges from a pileup with a "dislocated" finger.

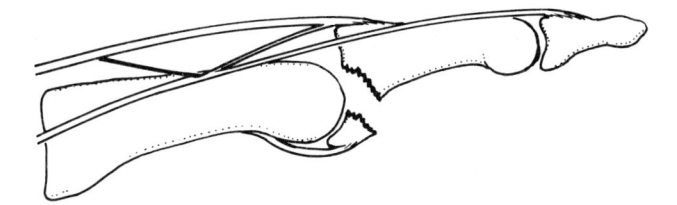

Figure 3-19. In coach's finger, the fracture through the articular surface of the middle phalanx dislocates the remaining articular surface of the middle phalanx dorsally. The pull of the extensor mechanism then maintains the dislocation and prevents easy reduction.

He presents the deformed finger to the coach who pulls the finger out straight and tapes it to an adjacent finger. By the end of the game the finger is so swollen that dislocation seems to have been reduced, but 3 months later when the finger still will not flex, a persistent fracture dislocation is confirmed by radiography (Fig. 3-19). Early treatment of this injury is less complicated and produces superior results. Delayed treatment requires extensive surgical reconstruction.

All finger joint injuries in which the patient does not have full motion of a joint should be x-rayed.

Bennett's Fracture. This is a fracture dislocation of the base of the thumb metacarpal (Fig. 3-20). Longitudinal force on the thumb fractures the bone and leaves a fragment of the articular surface of the metacarpal attached to a strong ulnar ligament. Pull of the abductor pollicis longus displaces the large metacarpal fragment radial and proximal. To avert the possible development of post-traumatic degenerative arthrosis, reduction to reestablish congruity of this joint is mandatory and frequently requires surgery.

Infection

Although antibiotics have revolutionized the prognosis of hand infection, improper treatment as well as delay in appropriate therapy can still be disastrous. Cure of an infection without surgical intervention can be achieved in only a limited number of cases. If the problem is diagnosed within the first 24 to 48 hours of onset, administration of high-dose systemic antibiotics and immobilization and elevation of

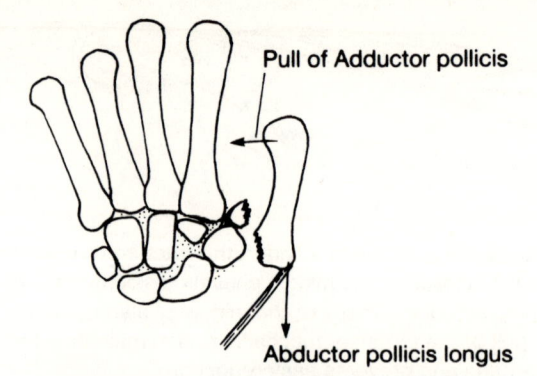

Figure 3-20. In Bennett's fracture, the fracture of the proximal aspect of the thumb metacarpal through the articular surface dislocates the metacarpal on the trapezium. The pull of the abductor pollicis longus maintains and even aggravates the dislocation.

the hand may be sufficient. After this period, success with antibiotics alone is unlikely because the many closed spaces in the hand permit early walling off of an infection and prevent antibiotics from reaching the site.

Simple hand lacerations should be managed with meticulous irrigation and appropriate débridement. More complicated wounds, such as open fracture, open joint, puncture wound, gunshot wound, and tendon laceration, merit the administration of prophylactic antibiotics. Patients with immunologic deficiencies, such as diabetes, and patients on cancer chemotherapy should also be treated prophylactically.

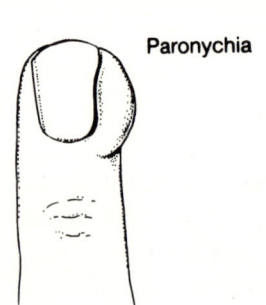

Figure 3-21. An infection of the skin fold next to the fingernail.

Injuries of the Hand 55

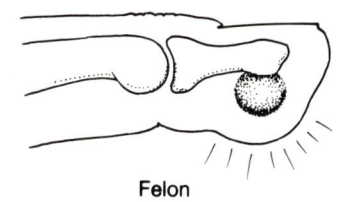

Figure 3-22. An infection in the finger-pulp tissue.

Felon

Paronychia. The most common infection of the hand, paronychia (Fig. 3-21) is an infection involving the soft-tissue fold around the fingernail. It frequently begins as a hangnail and usually is caused by *Staphylococcus*. The infection can spread all the way around the nail, in this case it is referred to as a "run around" infection.

Treatment involving warm soaks, oral antibiotics, and rest of the finger can abort the infection in its early stages. Later, surgical drainage is necessary.

Felon. This is a deep abscess of the distal finger pulp (Fig. 3-22), in which the finger pulp becomes red, swollen, and extremely painful. *Staphylococcus* is usually the offending organism. Drainage is usually necessary. If not treated early, the abscess can spread to the phalanx, causing osteomyelitis.

Suppurative Tenosynovitis. This is an infection inside the flexor tendon sheath that can cause extensive scarring and destruction of the tendon and thus merits prompt treatment. The infection usually follows a penetrating injury that introduces *Staphylococcus* or *Streptococcus* into the tendon sheath. It presents classically with Knavel's four signs: (1) fusiform swelling of the finger, (2) slightly flexed finger, (3) tenderness over the flexor tendon sheath, and (4) severe pain with passive extension of the finger. Treatment usually consists of surgical drainage of the flexor tendon sheath.

Chapter 4

Injuries of the Neck

David A. Labosky

The cervical spine consists of seven movable vertebral segments. A heavy skull at the top and a relatively fixed thoracic spine below make the cervical spine vulnerable to injury. The first and second cervical vertebrae are unusual. The first cervical vertebra, the atlas, is a ring without a vertebral body. The upright odontoid of the second cervical vertebra, the axis, protrudes into the anterior portion of the ring. Ligaments connect the odontoid to the atlas, providing stability but allowing considerable motion. The bodies of the remaining cervical vertebrae are smaller than the other sections of the spine, with the spinous processes of increasing length progressing downward from C3 to C7 (Fig. 4-1).

Stability of the cervical spine depends chiefly on the ligamentous structures and the muscles as opposed to the bony elements. Intervertebral discs are present between the bodies to serve a cushioning effect. The facets of the cervical vertebrae present a sloping surface that permits gliding in flexion and extension. Movements are possible in extension, forward flexion, lateral flexion, and rotation. The ligaments are reinforced by the ligamentum nuchae, which is a very strong, supporting structure.

The cervical spine is straight from an anterior–posterior perspective and slightly curved (in lordosis) from a lateral perspective. The muscles of the cervical spine may be palpated to determine whether they are in spasm, perhaps resulting in a deformity, or whether they are tight bands, producing a fixed contracture. The spinous processes are also

58 Trauma

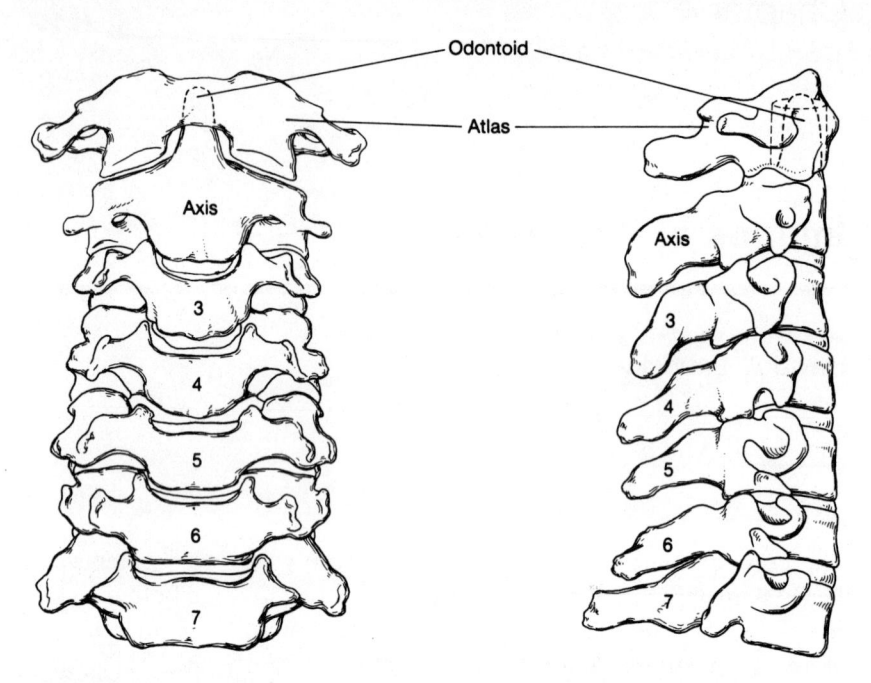

Figure 4-1. The cervical spine. Note that the atlas rotates on the axis in a configuration quite different from that of the other cervical intervertebral joints.

easily palpable throughout the lower vertebrae from C3 to C7 inclusively.

Examination of cervical spine range of motion should be followed by palpation for areas of tenderness, muscle spasm, contractures, and occasionally actual bony deformity. If there has been an injury, passive motion is contraindicated; only active motion should be tested. One must also determine the movement or position that produces local or radiating pain. Radiographic examination is usually necessary and should include, in general, lateral, anterior–posterior and oblique views, as well as a view through the open mouth. Lateral views in flexion and extension help to identify abnormal movement in the individual with instability. When evaluating these views, one must be very careful to observe the status of the prevertebral soft tissues and vertebrae, as well as possible loss of lordotic curve, and changes in the pedicles, the odontoid, or the disc spaces. Generally, a complete neurological evaluation of the upper extremity is also required.

Congenital Disorders

Klippel–Feil Syndrome (Congenital Fusion). This is an uncommon disorder involving failure of segmentation or formation of one or more vertebral bodies of the cervical spine. X-ray views may show bizarre anatomic relationships. Clinically, the patients show shortened necks with scoliosis.

"Wryneck" (Torticollis). This name is given to a condition in which the head and neck are held flexed to one side with a slight degree of rotation. The most common form of this condition is seen in a baby shortly after birth. Sometimes a slight amount of swelling is noticed in the sternocleidomastoid muscle, or this may be palpated as a very definite enlargement or "tumor." Reports indicate that the condition may be due to hemorrhage into the muscle or some injury, possibly during delivery; however, this has not been definitely established (radiographic examination is indicated to rule out congenital changes). The swelling usually disappears during the first few weeks of life but, if left unattended, the initially correctable contracture of the neck will become fixed. In order to try to preserve the length of the involved muscle and prevent permanent contracture, the baby's mother should be instructed in stretching exercises to correct the condition. Many times this home treatment is successful. In refractory individuals, resection of the muscle at a later date is indicated. If the condition is allowed to persist until later in life, contracture of other structures in the region and facial asymmetry occur.

Injuries

Soft-Tissue Injuries

Injuries to the soft tissues of the cervical region are usually caused by a sudden, sometimes violent, force. When the body is jarred violently, as in an automobile collision, the head, which weighs about 15 to 17 pounds (7 to 8 kg), may move rather suddenly. Such forceful movement can snap the neck and produce damage to the soft tissues, varying from a strain or stretching of the ligaments to a complete tear, which may result in a partial to total dislocation. Many of these injuries are now familiarly known as "whiplash injuries," a vague term meaning only neck pain, possibly of soft-tissue origin. When this type of injury occurs, the initial examination may not show much change and x-ray views may be essentially normal. Significant symptoms that localize the injury may not occur for a number of days. Sometimes changes are not seen until years later. Even though the x-ray findings are normal, with the patient only reporting pain and demonstrating muscle spasm, the patient deserves immediate treatment consisting of analgesics, rest, and support with a cervical collar. Such treatment is usually successful, with maximum improvement commonly reached in some months.

Sometimes ligamentous injuries are associated with a small avulsion fracture, representing a tearing-off of the bony origin, or insertion, of a ligament. X-ray views of such injuries require particular attention since the x-ray appearance of severe transient vertebral subluxations or dislocations can be similar.

Fractures and Dislocation

The spinal cord is enclosed within the canal of the cervical vertebrae, and the nerve roots make their exit through the intervertebral foramina on either side. The most common causes of fractures and dislocations are vehicular or diving accidents, a fall (steps), or a blow to the head. In the case of such injuries a rapid but very careful examination must be carried out to assess the neurologic damage and to establish a baseline for any future changes. During the initial examination the head and neck are usually protected by either light traction or sandbags and a lateral film of the entire cervical spine is made. After consideration of these findings, and the nature of any abnormal findings, a standard complete cervical spine x-ray series may be completed. Flexion and extension views are useful in evaluating stability but should be made only when indicated, and proper control must be maintained to prevent neurologic damage. Many of these injuries are associated with paralysis to a varying degree. Treatment often involves traction to the skull, by either tongs or a halo, or surgical open reduction and internal fixation.

Cervical Radiculitis

Lying down is the only position that actually rests the muscles of the neck. All the activities of daily living that involve upright posture (*i.e.,* sitting or walking) place the neck under considerable stress. Since the weight of the head is sufficient to buckle the cervical spine, active muscle contracture is essential for the head to stay upright. Under this continued stress, wear and tear of the cervical spine are inevitable with increasing age. This mechanical deteriorative process, cervical arthrosis or cervical spondylosis, can be seen in x-ray film in everyone by about age 35. It particularly affects the most mobile cervical elements, C4 and C5. Moreover the intervertebral discs between the cervical vertebral bodies may rupture out through their posterior annuli and put pressure on the cervical nerve roots.

Thus pressure on nerve roots can result from the inflammation and bony hypertrophy associated with arthrosis or cervical spondylosis and from actual herniation of cervical intervertebral discs. Pain may be felt in the neck but may also radiate down into the dermatomic distribution of these nerves into the shoulder, arm, forearm, and hand. Since the entire upper extremity is embryologically formed from a migration and coalescence of cervical elements, the pain from cervical spondylosis may also be felt between the shoulder blades. Therefore, when a patient presents with interscapular, shoulder, or arm pain, it is important to fully evaluate the cervical spine as the possible cause for these symptoms. The best screening test is hyperextension of the cervical spine for one minute. This will usually reproduce the upper-extremity symptoms if they are caused by cervical spondylotic or disc problems.

Tenderness over a cervical interspace will generally localize the area of difficulty. Limitation of cervical motion due to pain or remodeling of the intervertebral joints suggests arthrosis. Tenderness of a peripheral nerve and motor, sensory, or reflex loss in the upper extremities suggest a ruptured disc with nerve-root pressure. Although radiography will show some degenerative change in most older individuals, care must be taken when relating x-ray or mylographic changes to the symptoms. An intervertebral disc rupture may be superimposed upon an arthrotic interspace, or an arthrosis can be a late sequence of disc rupture. Treatment by cervical traction in flexion three or four times a day will usually relieve the radicular symptoms for 10 or 15 minutes. Occasionally disc excision, fusion, or arthrodesis of the intervertebral space is necessary. Extreme hypertrophy from reactive new bone associated with severe spondylosis may cause constriction of the spinal canal and the symptoms of nerve-root compression from spinal stenosis. This must be treated surgically. More will be said about the treatment of ruptured discs in Chapter 8.

Chapter 5

Sports Injuries

Eric L. Radin

Activities involving physical sports are associated with a high incidence of musculoskeletal injury. Peak performance requires close neuromuscular control of body segments. In the attempts to propel body segments at high speeds, to impart acceleration to a ball or other object, or to stop or block another opponent (in contact sports), the peak forces generated on the musculoskeletal components are very high indeed. This chapter will discuss how these forces are created and dissipated, and the causes, diagnoses, and treatments of some common sports injuries.

Forces on Joints and Periarticular Structures

The major forces acting on the joints are those created not by body weight but by the contraction of the muscles spanning the joints. These muscles are contracted both to maintain joint stability and to move joints. Of greater importance than the force *per se* is the force per unit area, or stress, on a joint. In fact, the most highly stressed joint of the body is the distal interphalangeal joint. Its contact surface area is small and the major muscles that span it (flexor digitorum longus and extensor digitorum communis) are very strong. Body weight makes up only a small percentage of the force on the joints of the lower extremity. Muscles about the hip must contract to stabilize the trunk and pelvis on the lower limbs. The force of this contraction is at least as great and frequently 2 or 3 times greater than the force of the body weight on the joint. The force on the hip joint in stance has been calculated to be about 2 times body weight and the force on the knee in stance about 5 times body weight. Because the joints of the upper extremities have smaller contact areas than those of the lower extremities, they are stressed equally even though the forces across the joints of the upper extremities are somewhat less than those across the weight-bearing joints.

In addition to the forces across the joint induced by weight bearing, one must add the reaction force resulting from the interaction of the body with the ground or some object. *In vitro,* articular joints will wear out under such forces; thus there must be some *in vivo* "shock-absorbing mechanisms" that spare the joint.

These shock-absorbing mechanisms can be both passive and active. The passive mechanisms include deformation of soft tissues (for example, the heel pad), cartilage, and bone. The active mechanism is the lengthening of muscles under slight tension. Consider landing from a jump. Upon landing, hips and knees are bent and ankles are plantar flexed. These joints are straightened out on landing and the muscles that span the back of the ankle, knee, and hip are stretched. The muscles act, when slightly contracted, as rubber bands, with energy required to stretch them. Thus, these neuromuscular reflexive actions spare the joint from the peak dynamic loads created by the activities of daily living. Failure of the reflexive neuromuscular protective mechanism can lead to injury of the musculoskeletal components.

The Role of Ligaments and Joint Capsules

Ligaments and joint capsules act to restrain joints from excessive motion. They do not direct joint motion *per se.* Joint motion is made possible by the two-part configuration of the joint itself. One can confirm this by studying cadaveric material. The knee, for example, will continue to rotate internally (tibia turning inward under the femur) with knee flexion even when all of the soft tissues, including all ligaments and capsule, have been stripped from the bones. This is a result of the conformation of the distal femur with a proximal tibia. The rotation is created by the unequal size of the femoral condyles. Since the medial is larger than the lateral, the tibia will have to move more medially than laterally, thereby externally rotating as the knee is extended, pivoting around the lateral condyle as it were.

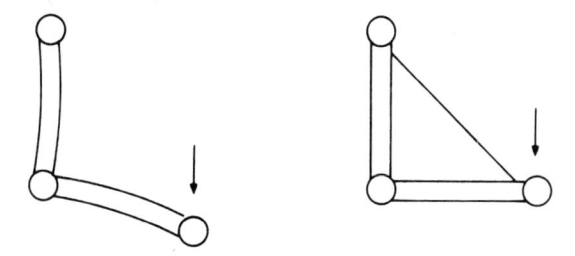

Figure 5-1. Weight on an outstretched hand is opposed by muscle contraction, which can significantly diminish the bending stress on the bones. (After Radin EL, Simons SR, Rose RM, Paul JL: Practical Biomechanics for the Orthopedic Surgeon, p 46. New York, John Wiley & Sons, 1979)

Rather than enabling motion, ligaments act as leashes in joints, to a greater or lesser degree depending on the joint. Most abnormal joint motions are usually prevented by appropriate muscular contraction. A loss of the anterior cruciate of the knee can be overcome by quadriceps- and hamstring-strengthening exercises. Thus, the ligaments and capsule are rarely stretched, except when the muscles fail to do their protective job, that is, fail to contract in a meaningful way at precisely the right time. A ligament might tear then as the result of an unexpected motion, a forced motion, a motion that occurs when the muscles have become fatigued from overwork, or motion beyond the scope of muscle control. The same can be said for the joint capsule, which also constrains the joints from excessive motion. Tears of joint capsule occur, but usually only from forced motions.

Nature of Damaging Forces

Damage to musculoskeletal elements is usually caused by a single excessive load (*e.g.,* the collision of two football players) or by smaller repeated loads (*e.g.,* repetitively pitching a curveball in baseball games).

Single loads can cause fracture, as sometimes happens when a skier skies into a tree or a football player falls on top of another. Fracture is an effective way to absorb energy, but requires a long period of time to repair. Muscles help to prevent fracture by limiting the potentially damaging tensile strain on the bone (Fig. 5-1). Thus muscle fatigue can be a significant factor in sports-related injuries, and sports enthusiasts should be warned not to play or practice when their muscles are tired.

Common Sports Injuries

Strains and Sprains

While there is no accepted precise definition for strain or sprain, both involve some form of tear or rupture. Obviously, force exceeding the resistance of the strength of a structure will tear the structure. Tears can be partial or complete. As noted above, the muscles surrounding a joint and joint capsule protect against excessive motion. Motions that surprise an athlete, that is, motions for which the muscles cannot be set, can force a joint beyond its normal range or in some abnormal direction. For example, sideways stress on the knee, if forceful enough, will tear the structures placed under tension trying to resist that motion. As another example, the ankle normally flexes and extends with some slight rotation built in. Twists of the ankle will pull on the ligamentous structures and cause ankle sprain.

A partial sprain of a ligament will heal if the remaining portion of the ligament maintains the continuity of the torn parts. Knee immobilization or periods of nonuse (crutches used to spare a sprained ankle) will allow the patient comfort but are not essential for healing. Strict immobilization is essential for healing when a ligament is totally torn. In this instance, if the torn ends are approximated, casting for an appropriate period of time will allow a natural repair. It is axiomatic that fiber-structure-to-fiber-structure healing requires 3 weeks and fiber structure to bone (*i.e.,* the bony insertion of ligament) requires 6 weeks to heal with adequate strength so that the joint can be used without fear of retearing. In both these instances we are assuming that muscle tone is normal and that the neuromuscular reflexes are available to protect the healed ligament from re-injury.

When a complete rupture of a ligament is suspected clinically, by the associated significant hemorrhage, swelling, instability when the joint is strained, or loss of normal alignment, it is difficult for the treating physician to know whether the ligamentous ends will be approximated after manipulative reduction. In such instances, surgical intervention is indicated to ensure approximation. The ligamentous ends can be trapped within the joint or under another structure or simply folded

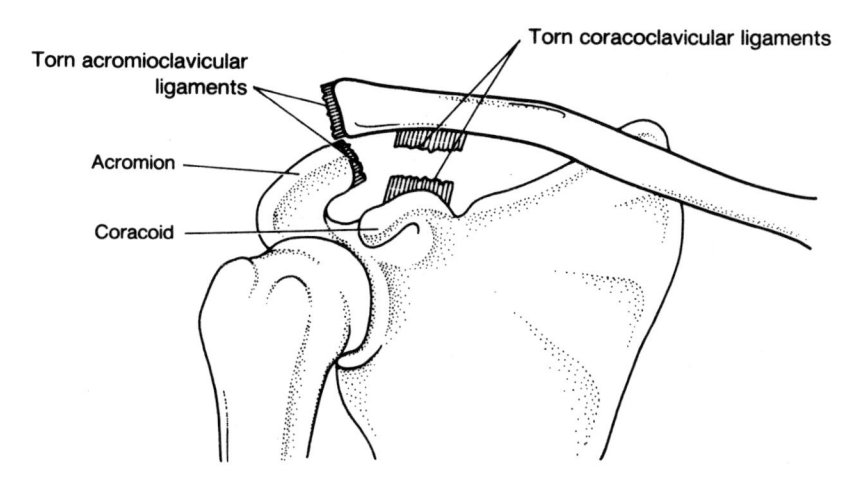

Figure 5-2. Complete acromioclavicular separation requires tearing both the acromioclavicular and coracoclavicular ligaments.

back on themselves. Failure to heal will leave the patient with chronic instability of that joint. Surgical intervention for completely ruptured ligaments has become common.

A case in point is shoulder separation or separation of the acromioclavicular joint. This is an injury common in contact sports and bicycle riding. A fall on the "point" of the shoulder produces downward pressure on the acromial process of the scapula tearing the ligaments that hold it to the clavicle. The joint is held together by two sets of ligaments, those running from the acromion to the clavicle and those running from the coracoid process of the scapula to the clavicle. There are various degrees of this injury depending on whether there is a partial tear of the ligaments, a complete rupture of one ligament, or a complete rupture of both (Fig. 5-2). If the ligaments are both intact, treatment can be symptomatic. If the joint is actually dislocated, while there will be a cosmetic deformity, function is not restricted except in heavy laborers and competitive athletes. The more common problem comes when the joint is only partially dislocated and a posttraumatic arthrosis can develop. Treatment varies from slings for comfort to open reductions with suturing of the ligaments to late reconstructions depending on the degree of injury and the expected activity level of the patient.

Tendons can also be ruptured in sports. This occurs, as in all structures, when the force on the muscle–tendon complex exceeds the ability of the structures to withstand the force. It is impossible to rupture tendons or pull muscles by contracting muscles because the Golgi apparatus in the tendons, when stretched, provokes a relative inhibition of muscle contraction and prevents "autorupturing" of a muscle. However, if a muscle is stretched while being contracted, the combined tensile forces can rupture its tendon. This most frequently occurs when an individual, doing one activity, shifts to another so suddenly that the neuromuscular reflexes cannot keep pace. Consider two persons lifting a heavy object. If one person drops part of the load, this may cause immediate extension of the elbows of the other person who now is trying to support all the load and has his biceps contracted. The result could be rupture of the biceps tendon. Another example would be a runner contracting the calf muscles at the time of toe-off. If he steps in a hole, his ankle will suddenly be dorsiflexed. The Achilles tendon will be stretched while the gastrocnemius and plantaris are being contracted, and the heel cord can rupture. If a tennis player is running toward one side of the court and is forced to change direction suddenly while the gastrocnemius and soleus are being contracted, heel cord rupture may again occur.

Most heel cord ruptures are simply ruptures of the plantaris tendon. Although such an injury may be uncomfortable for several weeks until the associated hemorrhage and swelling resolve, it is not incapacitating. However, true rupture of the heel cord, if it does not heal, is a significant functional impairment. Although it is possible to approximate the ends of the heel cord by plantar flexing the ankle and flexing the knee, this method of treatment has lost favor because it is unreliable; surgical repair is considered the method of choice. Because the gastrocnemius tendon is relatively avascular, it needs more time to heal than most other tendons.

Suture of tendons does not obviate the need for further support. A tendon may be strong when immediately sutured, but it will become weak over the next 7 to 10 days as the necrosis from pressure under the suture weakens the structure locally. The tendon will become strong again approximately 14 to 21 days after suture as healing takes place.

The substance of a muscle, like its tendon, can be torn when the muscle is stretched while being contracted. Again, this usually occurs when a person is performing one motion and suddenly is required to perform another. The muscles are rarely torn completely. A partially torn muscle is known as a *charley horse* and heals without treatment, although it can be very uncomfortable for several days.

If the physician has a choice in the type of immobilization to be used in treatment, crutches should be avoided. They involve both upper extremities and thus add to the impairment caused by an injury to a lower extremity. Patients prefer casts and strappings that allow more freedom of activity.

Tendonitis

Although a tendon can be traumatically pulled out of its bony insertion, a partial separation caused by smaller, repeated stress loads is the more frequent injury. Total separations are usually associated with avulsion fractures of the bony insertions and, in general, are diagnosed by clinical observation and radiography. In the case of partial separations, there are usually no x-ray findings and no well-remembered traumatic incidence. The patient may experience chronic pain whenever the muscle is used or the part is moved. This syndrome is called "tendonitis." The most common tendonitis is *tennis elbow*. This is a partial avulsion of the common extensor tendon or a partial tear of the common extensor tendon of the forearm. Common extensors act as extensors, or supinators, of the wrist. When the forearm is being forcefully supinated, the common extensors of the forearm are called into play to aid the biceps, the major supinator. In such a situation, extending the elbow, as in a poorly performed backhand swing in tennis, puts excessive tensile strain on the common extensor tendon and small rips can occur. Normally this would not be a problem, but making a fist or grasping will also call the common extensors into play to stabilize the wrist. These small tears of the tendon are never rested adequately. The pain on the lateral side of the elbow persists and is aggravated by activity. There is local tenderness over the tendinous insertion of the common extensor muscle group or the lateral humeral epicondyle. The healing process is characterized by chronic inflammation.

Treatment usually involves injection of a corticosteroid into the tendinous area. This anti-inflammatory therapy is generally curative. The small tear in all likelihood persists, but the associated inflammation around the tear stops, and the patient is no longer functionally impaired. Complete rest of the tendon is an unsatisfactory treatment, as it involves immobilizing the hand. In cases where the tear is substantial, surgical lengthening of the tendon is indicated since this takes the strain off the tendon and essentially lengthens the muscle–tendon complex. One should take care to differentiate common extensor tendon sprain (tennis elbow) from arthrosis of the radiocapitellar joint or nerve entrapments that involve the innervation to the lateral side of the elbow, as in cervical radiculitis.

Bursitis

Wherever a tendon goes over a bony prominence, as over the greater tuberosity of the humerus (at the shoulder) or over the greater trochanter (at the hip), a bursa, or fluid-filled sac, forms which allows easier gliding of the tendon over the bone. Excessive muscular force may cause minor trauma to these bursas. The supraspinatus tendon, as it crosses over the subdeltoid bursa, can cause a subdeltoid bursitis. The condition becomes chronic because in almost all motions of the upper extremity, the superspinatus is constantly used to help the rest of the rotator cuff muscles stabilize the shoulder. Treatment involves corticosteroid injection and occasionally excision of the inflamed tissue or the calcium deposits that can form within the bursa. The condition can be diagnosed by local tenderness over the bursa and by ruling out conditions such as cervical radiculitis.

Torn Meniscus

The menisci of the knee are washerlike fibrocartilaginous structures. Horseshoe-shaped, they cover the peripheries of both the medial and lateral tibial plateaus. The menisci move backward as the knee flexes and act to stabilize the distal femoral condyles on the tibia. The edges of the condyles are convex and are inherently unstable on the relatively flatter tibial plateaus (Fig. 5-3).

    The knee, because of its built-in rotation, requires freedom of the tibia or femur while flexing or extending in order for the menisci to move normally. If rotation of the tibia under the femur is blocked while the knee is flexing or extending, it is possible to catch the meniscus between the articular surface so that it will be torn. Wearing cleats or other shoes that provide significant traction with the ground inhibits tibia rotation. Football, as a contact sport in which players frequently have their feet fixed to the playing surface while their knees are forced into flexion, is a notorious source of torn menisci. The medial

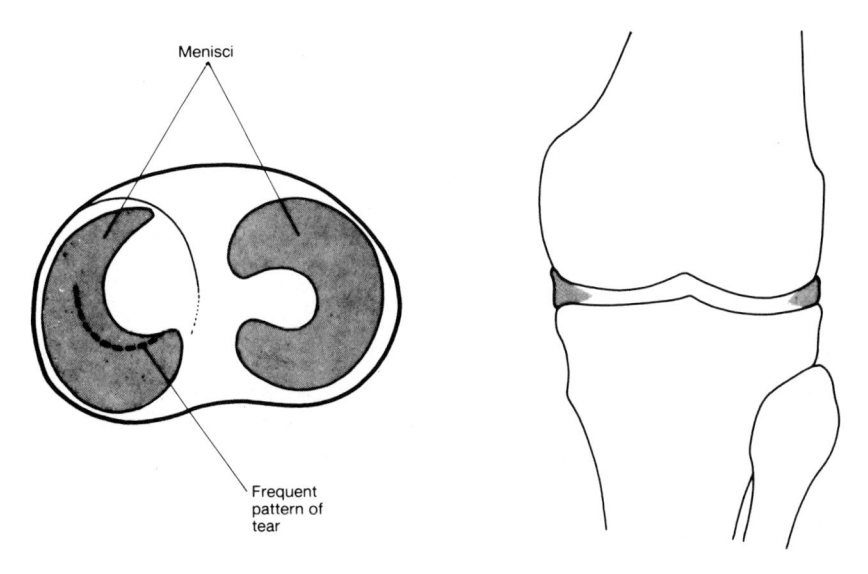

Figure 5-3. The knee menisci act as washers in the joint. The location of a common tear pattern in the medial meniscus is shown.

meniscus of the knee is more likely to be torn than the lateral because it is attached more firmly at its periphery and is thus more easily caught by an abnormal knee movement.

Diagnosis of a torn meniscus is made by history, signs of effusion and local tenderness, and either locking of the knee (inability to achieve full flexion or full extension) or a maneuver-instigated snap, produced by flexion of the knee while pressure is put across the symptomatic tibiofemoral compartment so that the torn portion snaps across the joint surfaces (*McMurray's test*). The diagnosis should be confirmed either by arthrogram (x-ray record taken with radiopaque dye instilled into the knee so that the dye fills the tear and makes it visible) or by arthroscopic examination. The arthroscope is a tube of small diameter that can be inserted into the knee. It contains a light source that permits direct visualization.

Treatment involves resuturing the meniscal tear if it is peripheral, in a vascular area capable of healing, or excision of the torn portion if it acts to block knee motion. Horizontal splits of the meniscus, which do not block motion since they do not cause catches or folds, are common and the result of simple aging. These need not be treated and should be considered an incidental finding on arthrographic or arthroscopic examination.

A total meniscectomy is rarely indicated but, if carried out, the postoperative treatment should encourage organization of the blood clot with subsequent fibrocartilaginous metaplasia to fill the space the meniscus once occupied. Such metaplasia is promoted by the avoidance of weight bearing and passive motion for a period of several weeks postoperatively.

Fractures

Sports-related fractures are usually of two types: (1) interarticular osteochondral fractures, caused by momentary subluxations or dislocations of joints where a piece of the joint is knocked off and (2) stress fractures of the diaphyseal shafts of the long bones.

The patellofemoral joint is the most common location for osteochondral fractures. The patella is relatively mobile and easily displaced. If it is subluxed or dislocated, it can easily chip off a portion of the distal femur. If the fragments remain partially attached, such fractures are referred to as *osteochondritis dissecans*. If the fragments become loose, within the joint, they can cause swelling and interrupt normal motion of the knee by jamming the joint surfaces and preventing full knee excursion.

Diagnosis of a "loose body" is based on the medical history, swelling of the knee, and persistent pain. Careful examination will sometimes demonstrate localized tenderness over an articular surface. X-ray films may or may not show the lesion. Tomography is frequently helpful if the lesion is small. Arthroscopic examination is indicated if clinical suspicion is high.

The treatment of osteochondritis dissecans is to pin or glue the fragment *in situ,* taking care not to damage the articular surface. The pins are inserted from behind. In growing children cast treatment is sometimes used if one can use the opposite side of the joint to hold the osteochondritic fragment in place.

Loose bodies are best treated by replacing and pinning them *in situ* or excising them. In young people the craters fill in or at least are asymptomatic. Excision can usually be carried out arthroscopically.

The popularity of jogging has made stress fractures or fatigue fractures a familiar occurrence. These fractures classically appear in military recruits who must make long forced marches during training. By their timely contracture, muscles that run parallel with the bones can limit the amount of bending stress on the bone. However, when the muscles become fatigued, the bones are unprotected and are subjected to increased bending stress. Hence fatigue fracture can occur. Such fracture, caused by a relatively low-level but repeated load, will slowly but inexorably extend across the bone. The patient complains of pain on activity. Fatigue fractures are almost impossible to see on x-ray film, and to make the diagnosis one needs the clinical suspicion, a history commensurate with such an injury, local tenderness, local swelling (a frequent sign), and a pyrophosphate bone scan that shows a localized area of increased radionucleotide activity. The treatment is rest. When the symptoms have receded, the offending activity should be resumed, but with proper muscle training. The patient should be advised not to indulge in any activity when the muscles are tired and no longer protective.

Traumatic Effusion

The joint capsule is lined on its inner surface by synovial membrane, which acts to secrete synovial fluid, the joint lubricant. The synovial membrane also acts as a "lymphatic filter" that cleans the joint cavity of debris. Trauma to the synovial membrane, if severe enough, can lead to a traumatic bloody effusion caused by rupture of the blood vessels of the richly vascularized tissue. The patient has a tense, swollen, extremely painful joint, which cannot be moved without acute discomfort. The diagnosis is made by history, physical examination, and examination of the joint fluid. Treatment is evacuation of the bloody effusion, compressive dressing, and splinting. This is carried on until the synovial inflammation associated with the injury has diminished, generally within a few days, but sometimes a week or two.

Less severe trauma to the joints can provoke a traumatic synovial effusion. This also gives a tense joint, referred to generically as "water on the joint," and makes it difficult to move the joint without discomfort. The effusion acts as nature's splint, a natural protective mechanism allowing the synovial membrane to rest while the microdamage is healed by the inflammatory process. If the synovial effusion is so great that it makes the joint tense and painful, it can be tapped. The tapping of synovial effusions that are from chronic causes, such as osteoarthrosis, is of little therapeutic value because the effusion simply reaccumulates. Synovial effusions left alone will gradually resorb. If they do not, the physician should suspect either that there is a chronic underlying cause or that the muscles protecting the joint are not doing an adequate job. If muscle strengthening is not painful, it should be tried for a few weeks before looking for chronic causes, assuming there are no bony abnormalities visible on film. Such chronic knee effusions are best treated with quadriceps strengthening. This maintains the integrity of the patellofemoral joint and in the face of weak quadriceps there are continuing chronic minor subluxations of the patella.

The physician should always consider infection as a possible cause of effusion. Infection can be ruled out by synovial fluid examination (see Chapter 6). Care should always be taken to tap synovial joints under sterile conditions; fluid obtained from any tap should always be sent for bacteriological study, to rule out the possibility that one is dealing with an infectious effusion and to rule out the possibility that the joint has been contaminated by a break in sterile technique during the aspiration of its fluid.

Part Three

Adult Orthopaedic Problems

Chapter 6

Reaction of Bone to Tumors and Infections

Rudolf K. Lemperg, Jamshid Tehranzadeh, and Eric L. Radin

Tumor and infection can affect bone. Because of bone's unique structure as an organ, its reaction to tumor and infection is a little different from that of the soft tissues. Tumor and infection do not themselves resorb bone or lay down new bone. What they provoke is an osteoblastic and osteoclastic reaction of the bone cells.

Bone as an organ has two main elements, cortical and trabecular bone tissue. Cortical bone, the osseous shaft or diaphysis, is relatively dense. Remodeling involves osteoclasis, which is slow and difficult in such structures; thus cortical bone remodels slowly. Trabecular bone, on the other hand, is surrounded by hematopoietic cells which are potentially osteogenic. Trabecular bone remodels much more quickly than cortical bone. In cortical bone, changes occur most rapidly next to the periosteum; periosteal new-bone formation is a common feature of a rapid cortical bony reaction.

Diagnostic Technique for Tumors and Infection

The critical diagnostic tool for studying part of the skeleton suspected of being involved with tumor or infection is x-ray (Fig. 6-1). What is seen by means of x-ray is bone formation and bone resorption. Most tumors and infections are radiolucent; they appear as "holes" in bone. They are distinguishable on x-ray films by the extent and apparent rate at which bone changes have happened. Judgment as to whether one

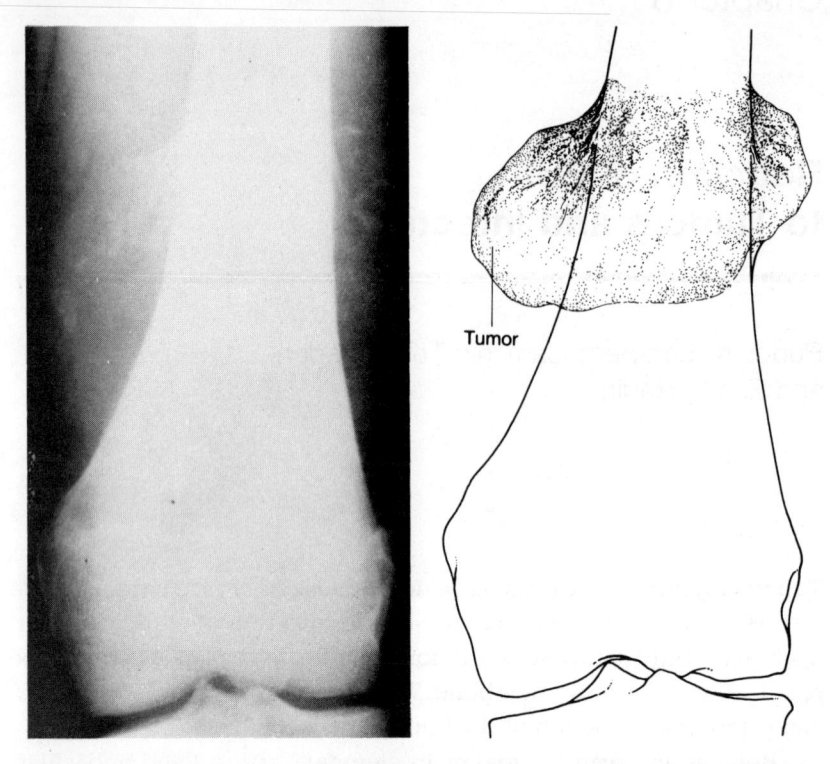

Figure 6-1. X-ray view of distal femur in a 17-year-old boy with an osteosarcoma. The tumor has broken out of the cortex and there is evidence of calcification in the soft-tissue mass which represents the extraosseous tumor. Note the new-bone formation in the adjacent soft tissues with aggressive periosteal reaction on both sides of the diaphysis.

is dealing with infection or benign or malignant tumor is based primarily on the degree and rate at which the bone responds to the pathological process. If the change is occurring rapidly, there is a less distinguishable margin around the lesion, that is, the area appears more infiltrated on x-ray.

Routine x-ray films of the involved areas should be accompanied by films of the same structures on the opposite side of the body. This enables the physician to compare structures and thereby detect minor changes. Such comparison is particularly important in the epiphyseal areas of the growing skeleton, where the secondary ossification centers may be misinterpreted as trauma or disease, but are really only patterns associated with active growth.

To truly judge perceived changes, one should always try to find x-ray films of the same bone taken at an earlier time. Since x-ray films are static pictures, views made over a period of time give much more information about the character and progression of any disease process in the skeleton.

X-ray views should also be made at different angles in order to obtain a three-dimensional view of the area of concern.

The physician should look for soft-tissue involvement, usually an ominous sign in bone tumors and one that is often present early in bone infections. This can be best done with a physical examination and a computed tomography (CT) scan. With its multiple cross-sections, the CT scan may also reveal the extent of the pathological process within the bone (Fig. 6-2).

Bone scan is an important diagnostic tool and an extremely sensitive screening method because it can localize all foci of ongoing bone formation (Fig. 6-3). It should be remembered that what is seen in a bone scan is bony reaction and, generally, not the process itself.

Bone scan measures pyrophosphate uptake by cells. Usually only osteoblasts, the cells associated with bone formation, will take up enough pyrophosphate to show a label on the scan. Bone activity persists after the acute reaction of bone has subsided, because in the healing phases the bone will remodel. Bone scans cannot differentiate between reaction of bone and bone remodeling, and thus should not be overinterpreted.

Arteriography defines the vascularity of a tumor and its soft-tissue component (Fig. 6-4). Actively growing tumors, particularly malignant ones, will show increased vascularity, enlarged and sometimes tortuous vessels, and an increased venous filling.

Tumors

Primary tumors in bone are rare as compared to metastatic tumors. The tumors that most commonly metastasize to bone in the adult are, in order of frequency, tumors of the breast, prostate, lung, kidney, and gastrointestinal tract.

Obviously, replacement of bone tissue by tumor will weaken the mechanical strength of the bone; the first symptom may well be a break. Since the bone is weak, the fracture will occur without the mechanical forces commonly linked to bone breakage. For example,

Tumor involving femoral shaft

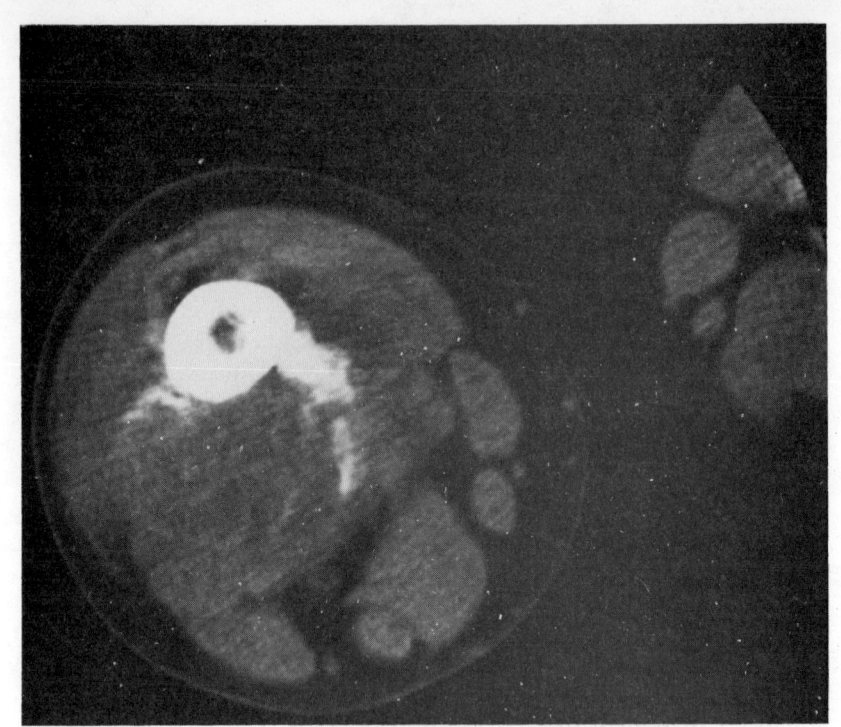

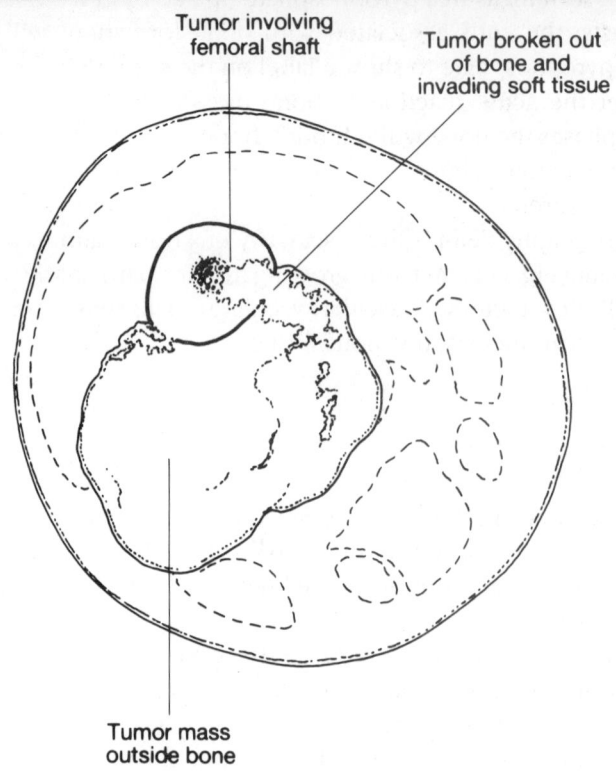

Tumor broken out of bone and invading soft tissue

Tumor mass outside bone

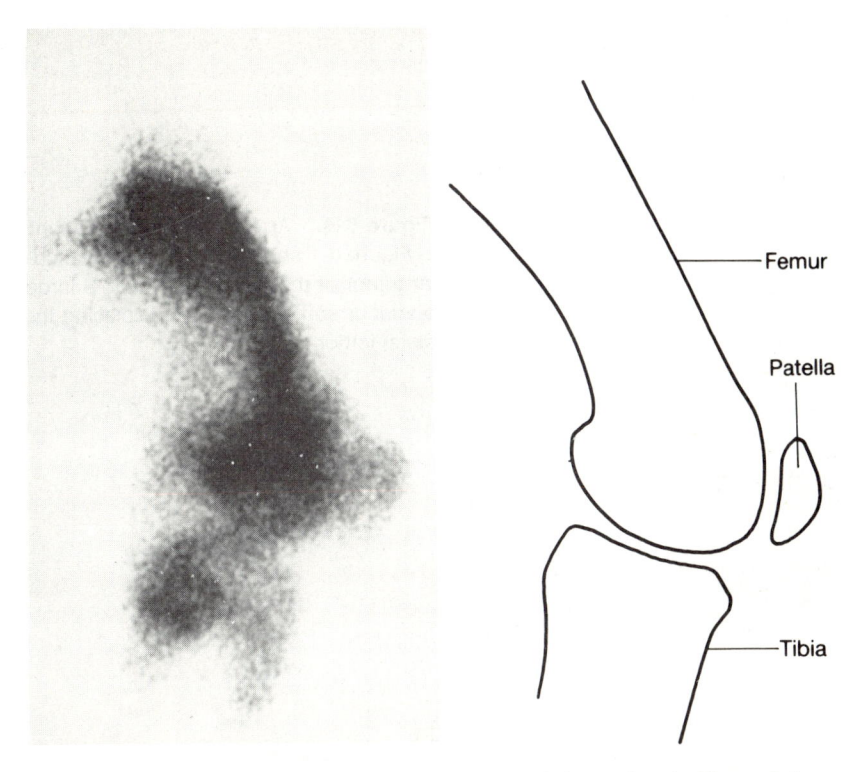

Figure 6-3. Technetium phosphate bone scan of the patient in Figure 6-1 shows marked augmented radionucleotide uptake of distal femur at the site of the osteosarcoma. Mild increased radionucleotide activity at proximal tibia is due to the localized hyperemia.

compression fracture of a thoracic vertebra might occur while the patient is putting on a coat. If a fracture occurs without reasonable trauma, the physician should suspect that he is dealing with a pathologic fracture. The most common lesion to cause pathologic fracture in the older adult is metastatic tumor.

Bone, the organ, is composed of a variety of tissues, each of which can give rise to tumors, either benign or malignant. Thus an easy way to categorize bone tumors is by their tissue of origin. Table 6-1 outlines

---

Figure 6-2. This CT scan of distal femur of the patient in Figure 6-1 shows large soft-tissue mass with new-bone formation in cortical bone and adjacent posterior soft tissues. Increased density in medullary bone suggests marrow replacement by the tumor.

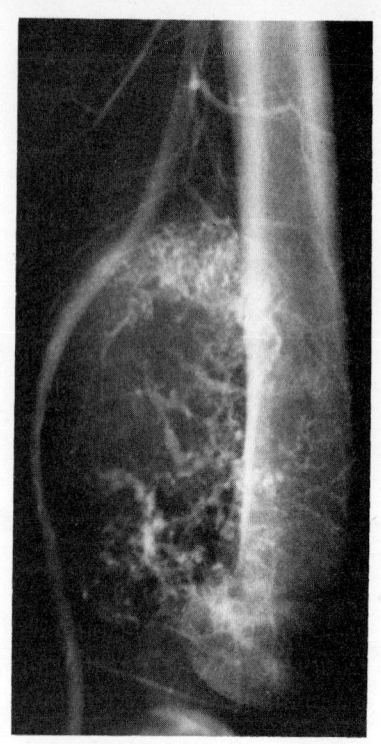

Figure 6-4. Arteriogram of the patient in Figure 6-1 shows a large hypervascular tumor of the distal femur with a large posterior soft-tissue mass displacing the distal femoral artery.

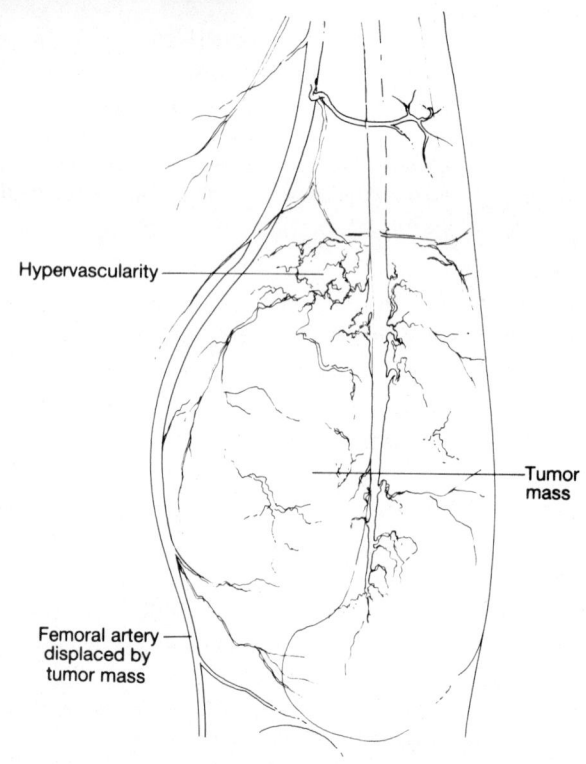

Table 6-1
Classification of Primary Bone Tumors

A. Osteogenic series
1. Osteoid osteoma
2. Benign osteoblastoma
3. Osteoma
4. Osteochondroma
5. Osteosarcoma
6. Periosteal sarcoma

B. Chondrogenic series
1. Endochondroma
2. Benign chondroblastoma
3. Chondromyxoid fibroma
4. Chondrosarcoma

C. Collagenic series
1. Nonosteogenic fibroma
2. Subperiosteal cortical defect
3. Angioma
4. Aneurysmal bone cyst
5. Fibrosarcoma
6. Angiosarcoma

D. Myelogenic series
1. Plasma cell myeloma
2. Ewing's tumor
3. Reticulum cell sarcoma
4. Lymphoma of bone
5. Hodgkin's disease

(Aegerter E, Kirkpatrick JA Jr: Orthopedic Diseases, 4th ed., pp 463–464, Philadelphia, WB Saunders, 1975)

Table 6-2

Staging of Bone Tumors

I. A low-grade tumor without metastases
II. A high-grade tumor without metastases
III. A lesion of either grade with regional or distant metastases

(Enneking WF, Spanier SS, Goodman MA: The surgical staging of musculoskeletal sarcoma. J Bone Joint Surg [Am] 62:1028, 1980)

the major benign and malignant tumors that arise from the tissues that make up bone as an organ.

For treatment purposes it is critical to know whether these tumors are locally invasive and whether they have metastasized. In order to clarify this, a staging for malignant tumors of bone has been devised and is given here in Table 6-2.

Stages I and II are further subdivided into intracompartmental (A) and extracompartmental (B). "Intracompartmental" indicates a lesion confined within the boundaries of a well-defined structure, for example, bone, joint, or fascial muscle compartment; "extracompartmental" indicates a lesion that originates in or has extended to areas that have no natural anatomic barriers to extension. The compartmental designation is irrelevant in stage III (metatastic) tumors. The staging system allows patients to be separated into high- and low-risk populations and thus facilitates planning of surgical management and adjunct therapy.

Effect of Age

The immature skeleton gives rise to quite different tumors, in general, than does the mature skeleton. For example, osteogenic sarcoma is common in the adolescent but rare in the older individual, except in patients with Paget's disease or multiple enchondromatosis (Ollier's disease). The latter condition is characterized by multiple cartilaginous rests in the metaphyseal area of the bone that arise from some generalized failure of epiphyseal maturation and can lead to late degeneration of a particular enchondroma into a malignancy. Paget's disease of bone is a localized or regularized lack of normal bony organization that is painful but benign unless it degenerates. For patients with these conditions, malignant degeneration of the formerly benign lesions is usually characterized by pain or the development or enlargement of a mass. Should such symptoms occur in these high-risk patients, it is important to consider malignancy.

Diagnosis of Tumors

In cases of suspected tumor, biopsy is required to make a histological diagnosis. Since errors in diagnosis can be made when nonrepresentative material is biopsied, it is important to differentiate between reactive new bone around a tumorous process and the tumor itself, which may or may not contain bone. Needle biopsy, done with radiographic control, has a reasonable chance of success in cases of metastatic tumors, round cell tumors, leukemic lesions, and infections. It may not be possible to obtain representative biopsy in solid tumors using a needle. A pathologist should be present at any needle biopsy in order to give an opinion (on the basis of frozen sections) while the needle is still in place as to whether suitable material has been obtained. If necessary, more material can be obtained from a different needle position. X-ray documentation of the site of the needle should be carefully made in order to avoid later uncertainties as to the precise location of the biopsy. Material should always be sent for bacteriological examination since infection can mimic tumor.

The physician must also keep in mind that certain "tumorous looking" processes can be representative of metabolic conditions. For example, fibrous dysplasias of bone may be manifestations of kidney or parathyroid disease. Other metabolic bone conditions that can be mistaken for tumors include rickets and scurvy. There are a multiplicity of malformation syndromes of genetic origin that may yield a strange appearance on biopsy. These are more properly identified by history and radiographic examination.

Prognosis

The prognosis of tumorous bone will depend, of course, upon the inherent malignancy of the lesion and the extent to which the tumor has progressed. Pulmonary metastases are most common in primary tumors of bone; CT scanning of the apical areas of the lungs is an important adjunct to plain x-ray when looking for metastases. The larger the tumor at the time of initial treatment, the poorer the prognosis. Bone tumors with localization around the knee and pelvis have a relatively poor prognosis. The more peripheral the tumor location, the better the prognosis. Malignant tumors of the hands and feet are rare. Histological grading of the malignancy of the tumor, based upon cellular pleomorphism, irregularity of the size of cells, and appearance of the stroma has not been extremely successful as a prognostic tool in bone tumors. Finally, the effect of a given treatment has to be evaluated using contemporary controls because historical control groups may have behaved differently. For example, the prognosis of osteogenic sarcoma became extremely poor in the 1960s and early 1970s, but has since improved.

Treatment

Surgical treatment has an important place in the overall treatment of patients with primary malignant bone tumors. In certain tumors, however, additional treatment is necessary. For example, in Ewing's sarcoma surgery can only be the adjunct treatment to primary chemotherapy and radiation therapy. As a rule, radical surgery to remove the primary tumor is still important in chondrosarcoma, osteosarcoma, and fibrosarcoma. It is less necessary, as noted, in Ewing's sarcoma, and it is not indicated in lymphoma, myeloma, and other round cell tumors. These are treated primarily with radiation and chemotherapy. Choosing the right therapy is often very complex because of the number of factors that must be considered, including expected survival, loss of function due to surgery, risk of complications from major prosthetic implants to replace radically excised segments, and interference by chemotherapy with the general health of the individual. There is a trend toward moving away from amputation and using segmental excision when possible.

An interesting attempt to influence osteosarcoma by interferon therapy should be mentioned. The rational basis for using this nonspecific, antiviral biological cell product was the belief that osteogenic sarcoma might have a viral etiology, which is true for certain sarcomas. Whatever the theoretical speculation, interferon has, in fact, in a minor series of cases, been shown to improve the short-term prognosis of a group of patients. Interferon does not appear to be the solution to the problem, but points toward the possibility of using the body's own defensive mechanisms against tumor. Whether or not further studies establish that interferon is indeed effective against osteosarcoma, the use of such nonspecific agents may become an important adjunct in our anti-tumor armamentarium.

Infection of Bone

Infection in bone can occur either by direct contamination, as in trauma, or by hematogenous spread. The metaphyseal areas of bone, particularly in children, represent a significant filter for blood.

Hematogenous infections are more common in children. They may be associated with infections in the tonsils, the respiratory tract, and the skin. The most common agent is *Staphylococcus aureus* (80%). Other agents include *Streptococcus, Pneumococcus,* and fungi, although tuberculosis and syphilis can also cause osteomyelitis. It may be very important to distinguish between gram-negative and gram-positive organisms; *Pseudomonas aeruginosa* must be considered especially in children. Sensitivity of the cultured organism to antibodies should be established in order to institute proper therapy as quickly as possible.

The possibility of tuberculous infection must always be kept in mind. Tuberculosis is more common in the United States than is thought. It frequently involves the ends of the bones and tends to spare the joint, although sometimes it can break through into the joint. The physician should do acid-fast stains on aspirates as a matter of routine.

One problem in the diagnosis of osteomyelitis is that 40% of the bone volume must be absent before radiographic evidence of diminished bone change is apparent, and in the early phases of acute osteomyelitis, there are no specific radiographic findings. These do not usually appear until at least 5 days or more after the onset of the infection. The diagnosis of acute osteomyelitis is thus made primarily on the basis of the physician's suspicion of its existence. Fever and other systemic signs of infection (local redness, tenderness, and swelling) may be present. When in doubt, early aspiration and Gram's stain of the aspirate are recommended.

With chronic osteomyelitis there is death of bone with osteolysis surrounding the dead bone (Fig. 6-5). The resulting pieces of dead

88 Adult Orthopaedic Problems

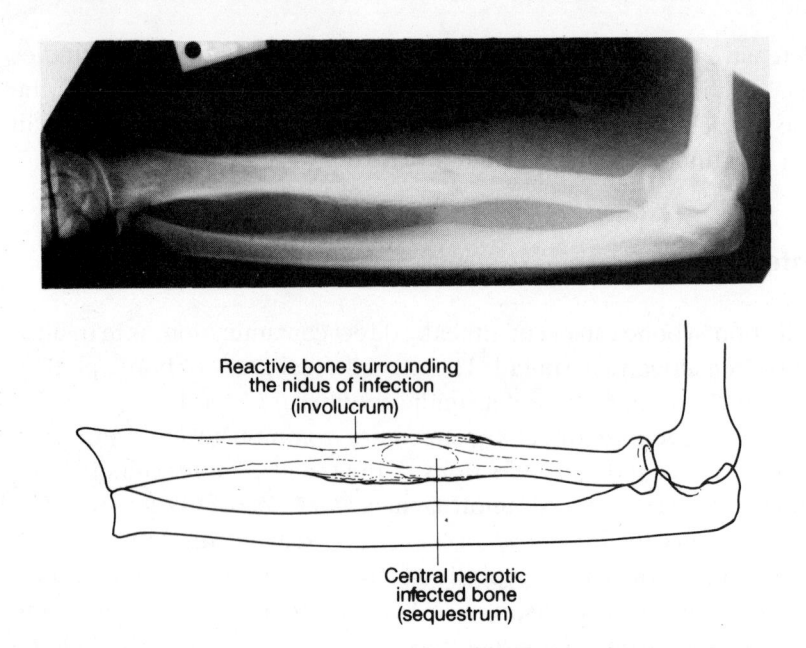

Figure 6-5. Chronic osteomyelitis of midshaft of radius shows bony expansion, irregular periosteal reaction, and a sequestrum surrounded by an involucrum. Note the irregular lucencies and endocortical bone resorption.

bone (sequestra) surrounded by granulation tissues can be diagnostic. The x-ray picture of chronic osteomyelitis is characterized by a combination of lytic within sclerotic areas of bone. Periosteal new-bone formation, often in several layers, is sometimes present, walling off the dead sequestrum. This reactive encasement is called an "involucrum."

In chronic osteomyelitis, drainage through a sinus tract may be evident. However, in some cases, the body may not respond with systemic signs and the diagnosis may require biopsy. Ideally, samples for bacteriological analysis should be taken from a piece of bone since in chronic osteomyelitis, there are frequently secondary bacteria in the sinus tract drainage that do not truly represent the deep bone infection.

A common diagnostic pitfall is incorrect antibiotic coverage. While the infecting organism may not be eradicated by the antibiotic, it may be suppressed to the extent that it will not grow in the culture medium. The result is a false negative report—that the infection is under control.

Treatment

The fact that infections in bone are so difficult to treat and to eradicate is directly related to the nature of bone and its circulation. In the soft tissues of the body, infection incites an inflammatory process that is highly vascular. New capillary beds can bring high levels of systemic antibiotic to the lesion. If the immunologic defense mechanisms are fully effective, infection can frequently be walled off from the rest of the body to suppress bacteremias. Abscesses can form and sometimes spontaneously drain. In bone infection necrotic debris rapidly clogs up the circulatory channels. Venous pressure rises and bone that is not directly killed by the increased pressure from inflammatory tissue is killed by the high venous pressures. Abscesses, if they form, will not drain spontaneously unless they are close to the surface of the bone. Moreover, the concentration of necrotic material in chronic osteomyelitis is an extremely attractive culture medium for bacteria, and it is not unusual for bacteria to lie dormant in bone for very long periods of time. Spontaneous recurrences of osteomyelitis are frequent. It has even been reported that infantile osteomyelitis recurred 80 years later in the same bone.

Treatment of osteomyelitis is, as noted, difficult at best and frequently entails surgery. If the surgery does not remove all the necrotic bone, the infection can recur. Treatment also requires higher than usual levels of antibiotics in the serum since it is likely that only a small percentage can get through to the bony lesion.

Acute osteomyelitis, with x-ray evidence of an abscess formation, should be initially treated with high doses of systemic antibiotics *after* a culture has been obtained. Sometimes, positive blood cultures will obviate the need for direct biopsy. If the patient does not clearly respond to treatment within 48 hours, surgical incision and drainage of the bone are proper.

If surgery is carried out after antibiotic therapy has yielded unsatisfactory results, the goal should be to drain and clean the lesion. A cortical window is made over the infection site, and curettage is carried out. This is followed with packing of the wound to allow it to heal by formation of granulation tissue from below. Antibiotic therapy should be continued until healing takes place.

Open packing of the wound instead of closure prevents necrosis due to increased intracompartmental pressure from edema and hematoma formation. Postponing closure a few days does not slow the ultimate healing time and helps to limit necrosis.

The problems in the treatment of chronic osteomyelitis are related not only to the bacterial infection but also to the extent of tissue damage in the bone and surrounding tissues. Since bacteria can breed in the remaining necrotic tissue over long periods of time, surgical débridement must be thorough.

Infection in Joints

Infections in joints (pyarthrosis) occur either following a puncture of the joint or by hematogenous spread. In the child diagnosis is easy to confuse with that of metaphyseal osteomyelitis. An infection in the metaphysis that is intracapsular may break out and enter into the joint, especially in the hip and knee. In the adult, the diagnosis is very difficult to make and usually depends on an extremely careful physical examination with pain elicited only on joint motion. All agree that it is important to make the diagnosis quickly and to treat the infection vigorously. Chronic pyarthrosis will destroy the articular cartilage and lead to postinfectious osteoarthrosis.

Intracapsular pressure produces distress and early dislocation. Diagnosis should be made by aspiration of the joint and study of the synovial fluid, including bacterial culture. White counts of over 100,000 per cubic centimeter are infections by definition. Acute crystalline arthropathy (gout, in particular) can mimic acute pyarthrosis and should be ruled out by searching for crystals in the synovial fluid.

In rare cases, acute osteomyelitis in children may behave identically to acute leukemia and thus be difficult to diagnose. Joint effusions following streptococcal or viral infections (*e.g.,* mononucleosis) might have similar symptoms, but often multiple joints are involved. Patients so afflicted never show high white cell counts in their synovial fluid.

There is not a consensus regarding the initial treatment of early cases of pyarthrosis. Some advocate immediate surgery while others prefer a 24- to 48-hour trial with carefully monitored application of intravenous antibiotics. If an abscess is already visible, clinically or radiographically, the latter treatment is not advocated. If the infection is in a relatively subcutaneous joint such as the knee, elbow, wrist, or ankle, it can be treated with systemic antibiotics and daily aspiration and lavage. Surgical implantation of tubes for lavage should also be considered. If these measures fail to rapidly improve the infection, open incision, drainage, and removal of infected synovium are indicated. Gram-negative pyarthrosis usually will respond well to intravenous antibiotics and rarely needs to be drained.

To understand the indications for surgery, one must keep in mind that surgery removes dead tissue and diminishes the pressure within and on the tissues and, thus, relieves pain, improves circulation, and diminishes the amount of necrosis. Limitation of necrosis is of special importance in areas where the circulation might be impaired and in epiphyseal growth centers, especially in the metaphysis of the proximal femur next to the hip in children.

The success of early antibiotic treatment depends upon having minimal tissue necrosis and adequate access to the site of the infection before further tissue is destroyed.

Chapter 7

Arthritis and Arthrosis

J. David Blaha and Eric L. Radin

Joint Physiology and Pathology

Diarthrodial joints allow the rigid segments of the appendicular and axial skeleton to move. Joints are specialized for low friction and for withstanding the significant forces exerted on them internally and externally.

The internal forces on the lower extremities are those created by muscles that cross and stabilize joints in order to support the weight over our feet on the ground. Without the action of these muscles we would collapse in a heap. In addition to balance, these muscles also provide the ability to accelerate and decelerate. External forces on joints are created by other muscles that allow the body to lift and move objects. Most of the force of the peak load is absorbed by associated structures before it gets to the joints. Thus, although the forces imposed upon joints at peak loading exceed that of the body weight by several fold, the joint is protected (see Chapter 5).

The size of joints correspond to the size of muscles. Thus, although the muscles of the upper extremity are smaller than those of the lower extremity, the pressure across the joints (the force per unit area), caused by internal and external forces, is equal.

The joint itself consists of modified ends of two bones covered by a bearing surface, articular cartilage, and surrounded by the joint capsule and ligaments. The joint is lubricated by a synovial fluid contained within the capsule.

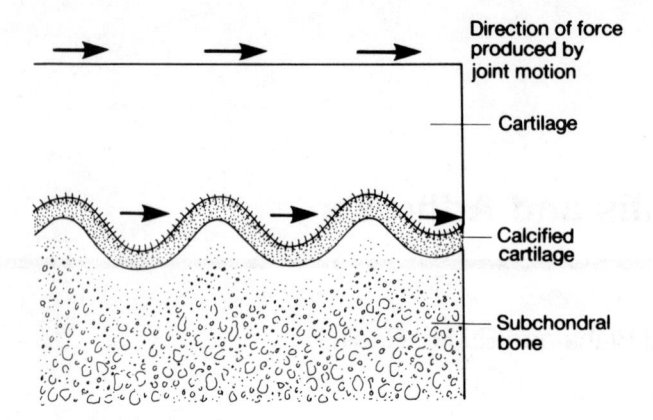

Figure 7-1. The undulations of the calcified base of articular cartilage convert potential shear stress created by joint motion, which would tend to separate cartilage from its base, into compression forces, which tend to hold cartilage onto its base. The anchoring of the articular cartilage is further enhanced by collagen fibers that traverse the interface.

Articular cartilage is a glistening white, very firm gel. Like all gels, it binds and traps considerable amounts of water, which it will yield when squeezed. The fibrous component of the gel is collagen, composed of a fiberlike molecule consisting of three polypeptide chains in a triple helical arrangement. Once secreted from the chondrocyte cell, these fibers are cross-linked to become a triplet. The individual molecules become arranged with each other in a precise manner and are further cross-linked to form collagen fibrils and fibers. The collagen at the surface of the articular cartilage is arranged in a skinlike, tangential manner. Collagen in the midzone of the cartilage is arranged in a fairly random pattern. In the deep layer it acts to bind the articular cartilage onto a transition layer between the bone end and the cartilage; this transition layer is calcified cartilage. The zone between the articular cartilage and the calcified cartilage is called the "tidemark" and is traversed by collagen fibers. The cartilage is held onto the calcified cartilage by interlocking collagen fibers and by the mechanical interlock formed because the interface is irregular (Fig. 7-1).

The primary component of the "ground substance" surrounding the collagen fibers is proteoglycan molecules. Each proteoglycan mol-

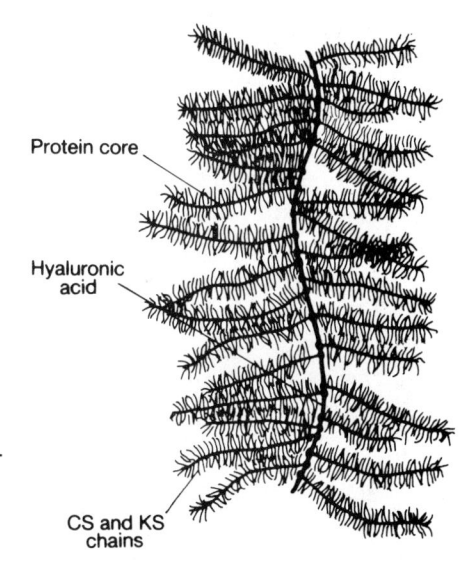

Figure 7-2. Proteoglycan–hyaluronic acid complex. There is a central backbone of hyaluronic acid with attached side chains for protein cores. The "bristles" sticking out from the protein cores are chondroitin sulfate (CS) or keratin sulfate (KS) molecules.

ecule is made up of a protein core surrounded by multiply repeating, covalently bonded disaccharide subunits. Ten to thirty proteoglycan molecules interact with the long hyaluronic acid chain and its associated disaccharide side chains to form these huge molecules (Fig. 7-2). Both the proteoglycan and collagen are hydrophilic and are capable of binding water. The proteoglycan is also very negatively charged because of its high sulfate content; it acts to bond water covalently.

The water in cartilage is both bound and trapped; trapped water is more easily squeezed out. Even strong dissociating agents, such as cesium chloride, will not remove all water from cartilage. (Cartilage must be put in an oven to be completely desiccated.) If cartilage is squeezed under physiologic load, it compresses by about 20%. The high sulfate content of the ground substance will create an osmotic gradient across the skinlike surface when cartilage is water deprived. Thus, when the pressure is removed from the cartilage, water from the joint fluid will be reabsorbed and the cartilage will swell. The collagen framework controls the amount of cartilage swelling. Articular cartilage contains no nerves or nerve endings.

The bearing surfaces of a joint are enclosed by a joint capsule and held together by ligaments. The outer layer of the capsule is composed of dense fibrous tissue; the inner layer is a highly vascularized, loose, connective tissue contiguous with deep layers of the lining layer, the synovial membrane. Although the synovial membrane is highly vascularized, it has few nerve endings. The capsule has multiple proprioceptive and pain-perceptive nerve endings. The lining of the synovium, three to four cells deep, includes cells that appear to be similar to macrophages and have a phagocytic function. The other cells in the synovial membrane have a synthetic function: they secrete hyaluronic acid, a major component of joint fluid. The synovium has numerous folds and a glistening, gravelly appearance.

Synovial fluid, found in the joint space, is a highly viscous lubricant composed of an exudate of serum with the addition of hyaluronate. Synovial fluid differs in composition from serum in that it does not contain certain molecules which would have difficulty passing through capillary walls because of their size and shape. The hyaluronate in synovial fluid acts to lubricate the synovial membrane as it rubs on itself and on cartilaginous surfaces. The cartilage surfaces, as they rub against each other, are lubricated by fluid that "weeps" out of the cartilage on compression, and by a glycoprotein-lubricating fraction, specific to the joint, which is found in synovial fluid.

The articular cartilage rests on the transition layer of calcified cartilage, which in turn rests upon a thin, bony shell that represents the articular end of the bone and is designated as the bony end plate or the subchondral plate. This is supported by a three-dimensional latticework of thin, bony plates interconnected by other plates and struts—the subchondral or metaphyseal spongy bone, also called "trabecular bone" (Fig. 7-3). The plates, or trabeculae, are arranged in such a way as to transmit the load from the cartilaginous surface and subchondral plate down through the articular end of the bone to the major central diaphyseal structure of the bone (Fig. 7-4).

Cartilage is sensitive to impact load and, when compressed, can crack. This cracking is called fibrillation. The peak loads created by musculoskeletal activity are lessened by motions of the joint, stretching of the muscles and ligaments that cross the joint, and deformation of the tissues themselves.

The synovial membrane is capable of initiating and sustaining an inflammatory response since it is highly vascular and contains macrophages. Because it has a rich capillary network within it, other inflammatory cells can migrate to the synovium, where they are then capable of enzymatic and antibody secretion. As mentioned above, the

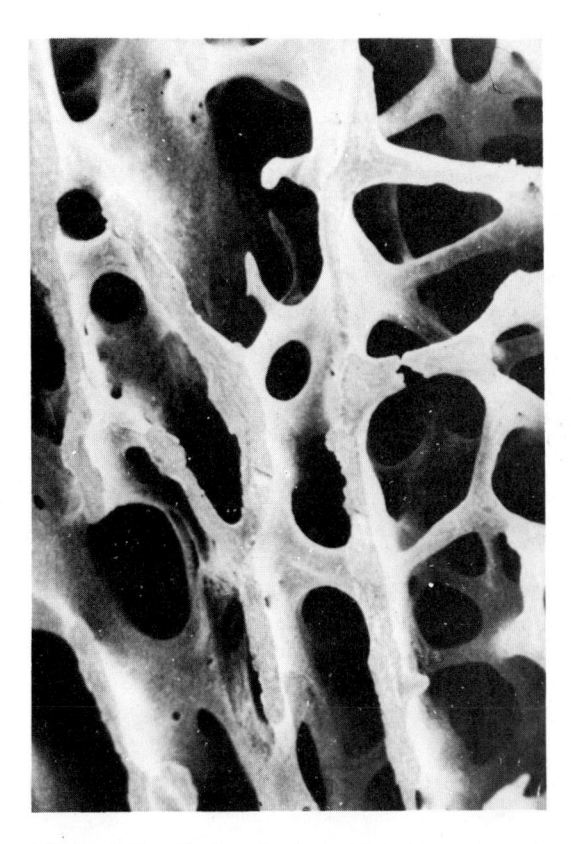

Figure 7-3. Trabecular (cancellous) bone is a three-dimensional structure, which is more evident in the photograph of a macerated specimen than in a thin histologic section where the trabeculae appear two-dimensional. They are really interconnected plates and struts.

cartilage is subject to fibrillation, and the bone that supports the joint is subject to microtrauma from repeated, poorly dampened impulsive loads, which can cause remodeling. The chondrocytes, the cells in cartilage that produce collagen and proteoglycan, are also capable of enzyme production (including lysosomes and kinins). Molecules within the synovial fluid, if small enough, can pass into normal articular cartilage. Once the cartilage has been fibrillated and its skin ruptured, larger molecules can pass within the articular cartilage and become trapped within its substance.

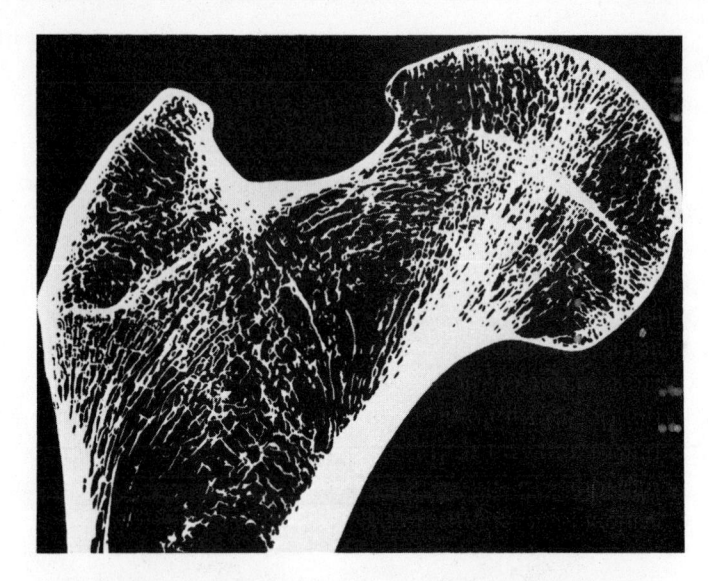

Figure 7-4. Trabeculae arranged to transmit load from the joint surface to the diaphyseal structure, in this case the medial cortex. (Thompson DW: On Growth and Form, p 232. Cambridge, Cambridge University Press, 1961)

Arthritis and Arthrosis

There has always been a certain amount of confusion regarding the distinction between osteoarthrosis (degenerative joint disease) and other forms of arthritis. Indeed, osteoarthrosis, as a separate diagnosis, was not distinguished until 1907.* The basic problem was, and still is, that all chronic synovitis leads to joint destruction, and all joint destruction provokes a synovial inflammation. From a practical and pedagogical point of view, we suggest dividing all joint afflictions into *arthritis,* primarily inflammatory joint conditions, and *arthrosis,* primarily mechanical aberrations.

Arthritis is commonly metabolic or infectious in origin. Infectious causes might include pyarthrosis (infection of a joint) or joint involvement as part of a generalized infection, such as the inflammatory arthritis associated with measles or serum sickness. In rheumatoidlike situations, joint inflammation is not clearly attributable to a particular

---

* Garrod AE: Rheumatoid arthritis, osteo-arthritis, arthritis deformans. In Albutt TC, Rolleston HD (eds): A System of Medicine, vol 3, pp 3–5. London, Macmillan & Co, 1907

pathogen and is chronic. The metabolically induced primary inflammatory conditions of joints include gout, pseudo-gout, and allied conditions. In these there is some metabolic abnormality, usually systemic, causing crystal deposition in the joint tissues with resulting inflammation.

Although pain in joints cannot come from articular cartilage, which lacks nerves, it can be traced to a number of sources, including synovial inflammation, stretching of ligaments, muscle spasm, and increased venous pressure in bone. The articular capsule surrounding the synovium is richly endowed with nerves; as the synovium swells, the capsule is stretched, causing pain. The inflamed synovium itself is a source of pain. Ligaments also contain receptors that signal stretching as pain. Muscle spasm occurs when muscles involuntarily contract to keep a joint from moving. Increased venous pressure anywhere in the body will produce pain; headaches, for example, are a result of increased venous pressure. In joints, the increased pressure probably occurs as a result of synovial inflammation. Inflamed synovium causes an increased secretion of synovial fluid, creating an effusion. Since the synovium is so richly endowed with small vessels, it probably acts as a filter or trap, sequestering various circulating antigens and provoking and focusing antigen–antibody responses and subsequent inflammation.

A diagnosis of arthritis can be made from history, clinical examination, and laboratory findings. The history is generally one of multiple joint involvement, usually symmetrical. As with most inflammation, there are few symptoms at rest. Involved joints are warm, swollen, and tender, and sometimes erythematous. Their motion is limited. Microscopic examination of joint fluid aspirates will show an increased white count and, if present, crystals or bacteria. X-ray views in the early phases are unremarkable except for effusion. In the later stages, the cartilage may be digested by inflammatory enzymes and radiographic examination will reveal loss of joint space. The inflammatory synovium may actually invade the cartilage and then the subchondral bone, causing bony erosion, formation of cysts, and collapse of the joint surface. There is usually no new-bone formation (Fig. 7-5).

Arthrosis (osteoarthrosis) results basically from the mechanical wear and tear of a joint caused by a localized increase in stress (stress concentration). Stress concentrations can be the result of congenital, developmental, or traumatic effects. In these situations one speaks of "anatomically imperfect" joints. An example of a congenital cause

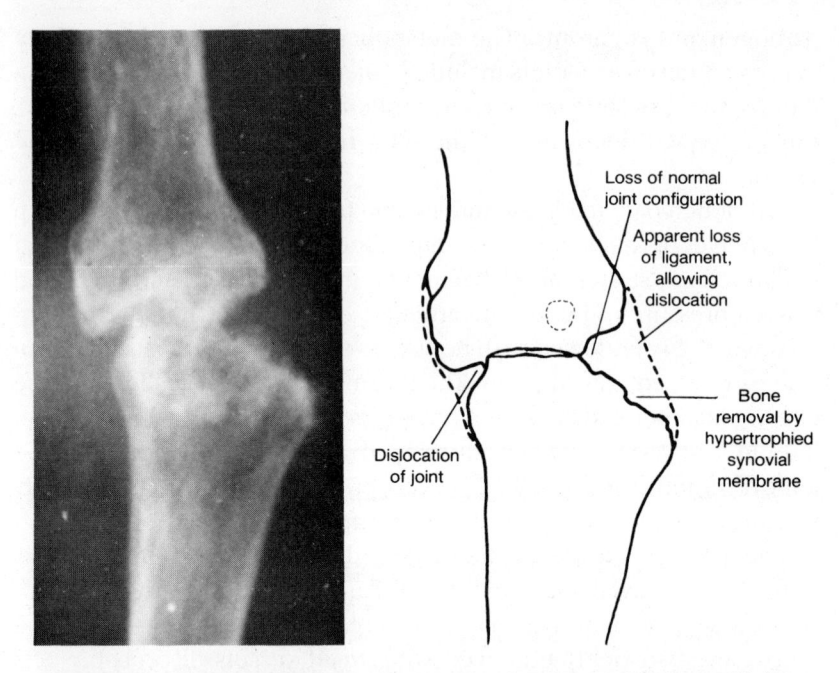

Figure 7-5. Advanced rheumatoid arthritis of metacarpophalangeal joint of index finger. Note the bony erosive changes, subchondral cysts, and deformities. Soft-tissue swelling around this joint represents thick and inflamed synovial tissue.

would be a congenitally dislocated hip; a slipped capital femoral epiphysis is a developmental abnormality. An example of traumatically caused arthrosis is an intra-articular fracture that has destroyed part of the articular surface. There is also believed to be an idiopathic subset of arthrosis perhaps related to the primary changes in the subchondral bone. In anatomically normal joints, stress is increased when the applied loads from activities of daily living overwhelm the normally occurring "shock-absorbing" mechanisms, which act to dampen peak forces and protect the joints. The major protective mechanism is thought to be the reflex stretching of muscles under slight tension (see Chapter 5).

Once the cartilage breaks down, free-sulfated proteoglycans from the matrix are liberated into the synovial cavity. These free-sulfated proteoglycans provoke an inflammatory synovitis. Thus, inflammation follows arthrosis. It should be noted, also, that mechanical breakdown follows arthritis in joints that have been sufficiently damaged by a primary inflammatory process.

The patient with arthrosis commonly presents with a history of a preexisting congenital, developmental, or traumatic diagnosis. Sometimes, however, there is no obvious cause. The joint complaints are usually limited to one joint or a group of joints (*e.g.,* both knees) and are characterized by pain, limitation of motion, and joint effusion. The hallmark of arthrosis is the production of new bone around the joint margins as lips, spurs, and osteophytes (Fig. 7-6). These tend to limit joint motion. There is also a profound stiffening of the subchondral and metaphyseal bone. In some arthrotic joints, osteolytic and osteoblastic processes (bone resorptive and formative processes) occur simultaneously. Generalized nodal osteoarthrosis, an intense inflammatory affliction of joints which causes severe joint destruction, should be considered an arthritis with a secondary arthrosis.

Treatment of Arthritis and Arthrosis

Pain is the primary indication for surgical treatment of arthritis and arthrosis. Occasionally, though, patients will limit their function to such a degree that they no longer complain of pain, only of decreased function. Limited function results in shortened resting length of muscle; this and scarring can result in contracture. A joint with a contracture is not always painful, but will definitely have decreased function because of the more limited range of motion. Thus, patients who are candidates for surgical treatment will have some combination of pain, loss of function, and joint contracture.

Since there is considerable risk associated with surgical therapy, other forms of appropriate therapy should be exhausted before surgery is decided upon.

Medicine aimed at reducing inflammation in arthritis includes aspirin, nonsteroidal anti-inflammatory agents, and immunosuppressive drugs, such as methotrexate, gold, penicillamine, and steroids. "Chemical synovectomy" using radioactive substances injected into the joint to reduce the mass of inflamed synovium has been tried with some success. The most common arthritis is rheumatoid arthritis. When therapy is started early in the course of rheumatoid arthritis, medical

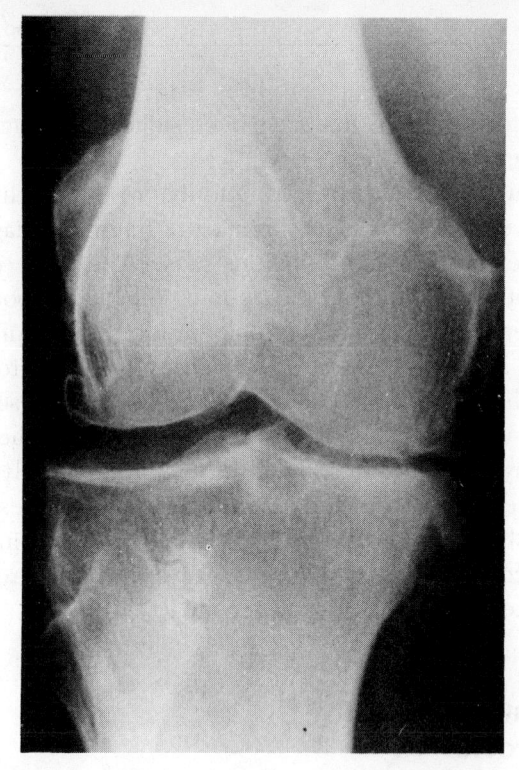

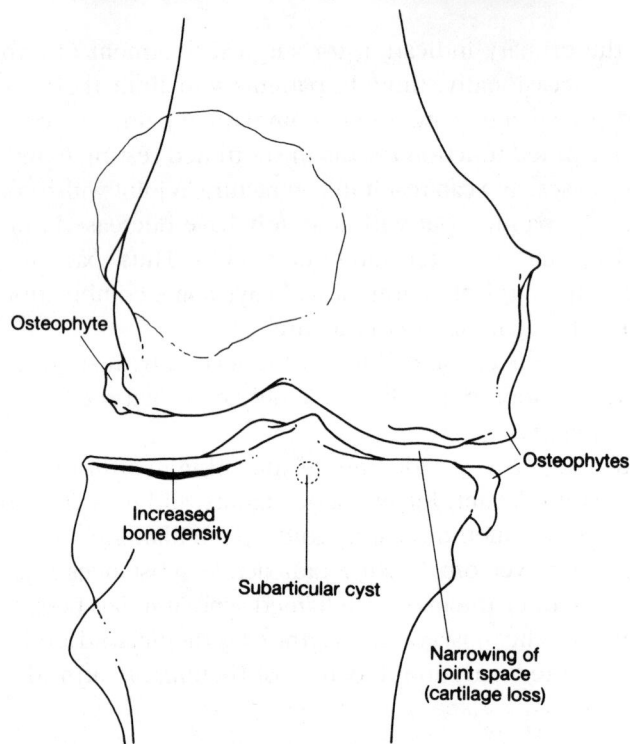

Osteophyte

Osteophytes

Increased bone density

Subarticular cyst

Narrowing of joint space (cartilage loss)

management is quite reliable for reducing symptoms and avoiding surgery.

Medical treatment for arthrosis is not as successful since the cause of symptoms is less clearly understood; however, increased venous pressure within the markedly remodeled subchondral and metaphyseal bone has been shown to cause much of the pain. The nonsteroidal anti-inflammatory drugs (possibly working through their inhibition of prostaglandin synthesis) seem to be successful, probably helping to suppress the secondary arthritis (synovial inflammation). As time passes, if nothing changes to halt the joint deterioration and subchondral bone remodeling and if stiffening intensifies, drugs become less and less effective in relieving symptoms.

Physical therapy to increase range of motion and strengthen muscles in joint disease is helpful because immobilization of the joint will lead to contracture and loss of range of motion. The only time immobilization is appropriate is during acute stages of synovitis.

When surgery is finally selected as the method of treatment, the following general principles should be borne in mind:

1. If the patient's main source of discomfort (and loss of function) is from an inflammatory problem, surgery should be aimed at reducing inflammation.
2. If the patient's main source of discomfort (and loss of function) is from a mechanical problem, surgery should be aimed at reducing the mechanical overload or maldistribution of load.
3. The best operation is the least radical one that will still provide the patient with adequate control of the symptoms; the physician should disturb or remove the smallest amount of tissue possible.

Synovectomy

Although inflammatory disease usually responds to medical treatment, occasionally a joint will remain inflamed with a boggy synovitis. In this case a synovectomy (removal of the synovium) may be appropriate.

Figure 7-6. Advanced osteoarthrosis of knee joint. Note hypertrophic osteophyte formation at proximal tibia and distal femur. The medial knee-joint space is markedly narrowed.

While synovectomy can be effective in reducing the cartilage damage caused by synovial inflammation, the primary reason to consider surgery is pain relief. Because synovectomy only relieves pain, it is not indicated for patients displaying obvious joint destruction. Synovectomy can frequently leave the patient with a slight decrease in range of motion; it is relatively rare to find patients with increased range of motion after operation. Thus, to be a candidate for synovectomy a patient should have at least a functional range prior to operation. The knee is the most common joint for synovectomy, followed by the elbow and the ankle.

Osteotomy and Other Pressure-Relieving Operations

The study of the mechanics of the body and the response of tissues to the forces on them is called *biomechanics*. Friedrich Pauwels, the "father" of orthopaedic biomechanics, proposed a logical way to think about the forces across joints, and operations for realigning these forces so that concentrations can be avoided.*

For osteoarthrosis of joints (*i.e.,* degenerative arthritis), operations have been devised to attempt to redistribute (presumably) unacceptably high joint pressures (too much force over too small an area). Osteotomies (Fig. 7-7A), tibial tubercle advancements (Fig. 7-7B), and greater trochanteric advancements (Fig. 7-7C) are examples of operations designed to redistribute the forces generated within the musculoskeletal system.

Operations for the relief of pressure are undertaken less often in the United States than in Europe, where many surgeons believe that if the operation is carried out with the proper degree of precision, it will yield long-term success. Indeed, it has been shown that there can be actual regeneration of cartilaginous tissue (albeit more fibrocartilaginous than hyaline) when forces across joints are minimized.

There has been less success with these operations in the United States than in Europe. In fact, osteotomy and "hanging hip" operations have fallen into disfavor with many orthopaedists in the United States. American surgeons claim that their European colleagues overemphasize the good results while the European surgeons claim that the

---

* Pauwels F: The Biomechanics of the Locomotor Apparatus. Berlin, Springer-Verlag, 1980

Arthritis and Arthrosis 105

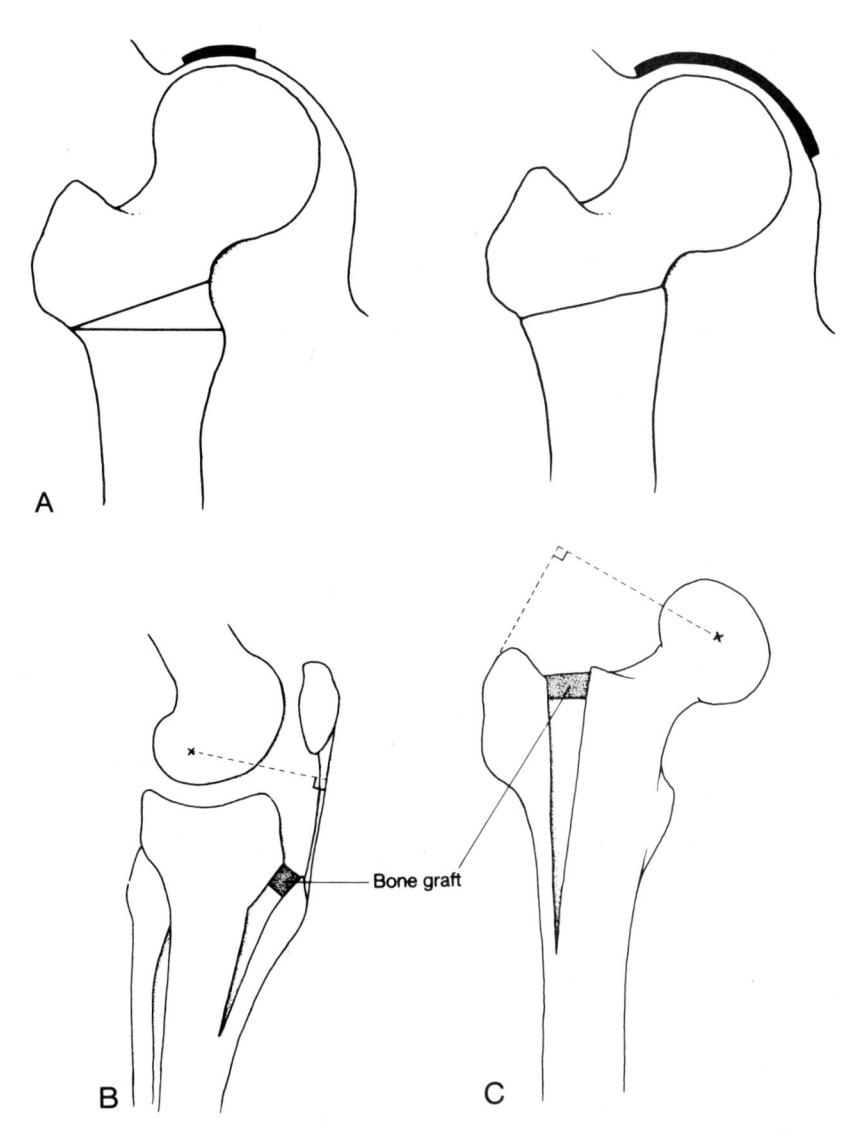

Figure 7-7. *A:* One of many osteotomies, this one is done for osteoarthrosis. Removal of the wedge, shown in the top left drawing, enlarges the weight-bearing area. Tibial tubercle advancement (*B*) and greater trochanteric advancement (*C*) are examples of surgically moving the insertion of a muscle to increase the lever arm and to decrease the joint reaction force.

Americans do not do the operation correctly. The controversy may be simply one of differing expectations.

Osteotomy is an operation designed to cut the bone and to fix it into an alignment that relieves pressure in the joint. This is accomplished by decreasing the overall resultant force on the joint or by increasing the surface area available to carry that force, or by accomplishing both. Osteotomy, an operation of many varieties that changes bone alignment, is most appropriate at the hip and the knee, and is seldom done for arthrotic conditions about any other joint. The "hanging hip" is an operation that partially cuts, and thereby weakens, the primary motors about the hip joint. By reducing the amount of force that can be generated by these muscles, that amount of reaction force in the joint is reduced. The operation is indicated only about the hip joint. All but abandoned in this country, hanging hip operation is still used by some in Europe; to date it has not found a place in the hands of most orthopaedists.

Osteotomy is indicated in patients who have mechanical disease of a joint directly related to a deformity of the joint. Frequently, the reaction of the subchondral bone of a joint can give a clue as to the abnormal concentration of forces and thus help in the design of an operation.

The operation is contraindicated in arthritis. Osteotomy is more successful early in the course of arthrosis and can be most rewarding in patients who show only mild radiographic changes but who are beginning to complain of pain. Surgeons disagree as to the severity of disease that can be treated with osteotomy. Because of problems that exist with joint replacement, osteotomy is frequently indicated for younger patients who wish to remain active despite severe arthrotic change in a joint.

Arthrodesis

Arthrodesis is an operative treatment for joint disease (Fig. 7-8). The operation essentially removes both joint surfaces and places surfaces of cancellous bone together in such a manner that fracture-healing mechanisms are called into play and the bone surfaces are firmly united; the joint no longer exists. The procedure has the advantage of absolutely removing pain (if there is no joint, there is no joint pain). Bone responds to Wolff's law across an arthrodesis, that is, the bone gets

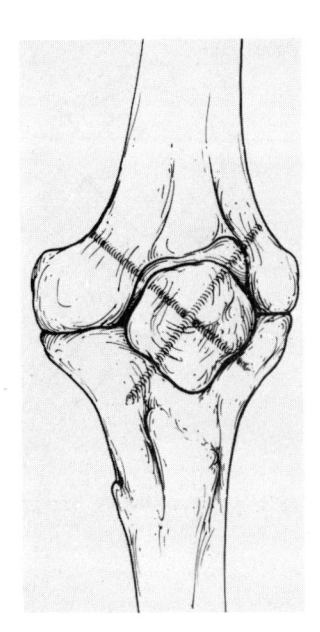

Figure 7-8. Obliteration of the knee joint by removing the articular cartilage, setting the kneecap into the front of the tibio-femoral joint, and holding the fusion immobilized with the cross screws. (Evarts CM (ed): Surgery of the Musculoskeletal System, vol 3, p 7:326. New York, Churchill Livingstone, 1983, by permission)

stronger as it is used more; for this reason a solid arthrodesis can be expected to stand up to heavy work, a definite advantage over joint replacement. But this advantage comes at the risk of causing degeneration of adjacent joints because the joints above and below the arthrodesis are made to function in the place of the arthrodesed joint. Patients frequently find the clumsiness of an arthrodesed joint to be a significant disadvantage. Its primary indication is in young patients with mechanical (usually post-traumatic) arthrosis of a single joint. It is generally contraindicated in patients with severe inflammatory disease because the joints above and below may become severely involved as well. Arthrodesis is done frequently in the case of rheumatoid arthritis of the wrist.

Total Joint Replacement

When all other treatment fails or is inappropriate, a total joint replacement can be considered. A joint replacement is termed a "total" when it resurfaces both sides of the joint with implants fixed to the skeleton; joint motion occurs between these implants (Fig. 7-9).

Because of the rather ubiquitous nature of arthrosis and arthritis

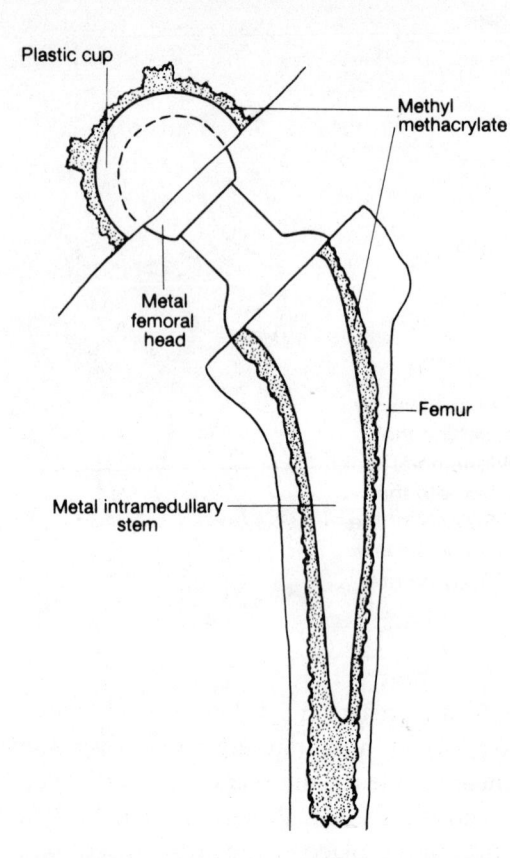

Figure 7-9. A schematic representation of total hip replacement. The proximal femur and femoral head have been replaced by a stemmed prosthesis implanted in the femoral shaft with methyl methacrylate "bone cement." The acetabulum has been replaced by a plastic cup, also held in place by the cement.

and the severely disabling pain related to these conditions, surgeons searched for many years for an appropriate replacement joint. Many ingenious solutions to the problem were tried, including implantation of bovine cartilage and Pyrex glass cups, and fascia lata interposition. In the early 1950s femoral head replacements were developed, consisting of a metallic ball (of the appropriate size for the acetabulum) attached to a metal stem that was placed into the shaft of the femur. This hemi-arthroplasty (resurfacing only one side of the joint surface) was relatively successful and became increasingly popular in the treatment of femoral neck fracture and aseptic necrosis of the femoral head. Frequently, however, these femoral head replacements were associated with progressive acetabular surface degeneration leading to pain and migration of the femoral head into the pelvis.

In the late 1950s in the north of England, Charnley, later to be Sir

John Charnley, began work to develop a joint replacement that would resurface both sides of the joint. To minimize the effects of prosthesis-to-bone motion, Sir John made two contributions which have made modern joint replacement possible. First, he developed a metal-against-plastic bearing surface that provides for a low-friction bearing. After first proving that Teflon would not work as this metal–plastic bearing, Charnley tested surgical metal against polyethylene. Today these surfaces stand as the most commonly used artificial replacement surfaces. However, recent reports from Europe, where patient follow-up has been more extensive than in the U.S., suggest that polyethylene hip sockets begin to deteriorate after 17 to 20 years. Other, perhaps longer-tolerated materials are being tested.

Sir John's second contribution was the introduction of methyl methacrylate (commonly known as Plexiglas or Lucite) as a grouting agent to hold a prosthesis in place. Methyl methacrylate is a self-curing polymer that is biologically well tolerated. It has been used for years in the field of dentistry for the fabrication of dentures. When mixed into a paste, the material can be forced into a cavity in bone where it will harden to form an exact negative cast of the bone. The early fit is so good that the bone must virtually be shattered to remove the acrylic "cement." There is, however, no direct chemical bonding of cement to bone.

Joint replacement using methyl methacrylate began in the United States about 1968; initial results were outstandingly successful. With time, however, these results became somewhat "less good." Even though the expected wear-life of metal against polyethylene as a bearing appears to be in excess of 10 to 15 years, joints began to "fail" with an alarming frequency only 5 to 10 years after the operation. The cement-to-bone bond seemed to loosen with time. Some of the loosening led to breaking of components and some merely to painful joints. Laboratory research into the reasons for loosening has implicated bony remodeling adjacent to the "cement" as a consequence of the implantation of "stiff" prosthetic components into bone; that is, stress sparing (see Chapter 2) is seen as the major factor in aseptic loosening. As a result, new prosthetic designs, new materials, and new means of handling the cement (and even avoiding it altogether) have been developed. Thus, it is very difficult to get a clear statistic as to how well total joint replacements are surviving today.

For total hip operations done in the United States with a follow-up of 10 years or more, it appears that about 30% of femoral components either have required revision or appear radiographically to have "impending" loosening. In published reports, radiographic evidence of some failure of the cement-to-bone contact appears in more than 90% of cases with follow-up of 10 years or more. Changes in technique have led to results that are apparently better at 5 years, but more time is necessary to assess the 10-year results with newer techniques. Whenever a new design or technique is used, the 10-year-result clock must be reset.

Younger patients and heavier patients seem to loosen prostheses more rapidly than older and lighter patients. In general, there is some product of *function* times *time,* which, when a critical point is reached, leads to loosening (L = F × T). *Function* can be body weight or heavy work. *Time,* of course, is related to the age of the patient. If a joint replacement is done in a patient who will not do heavy work, most experts will agree that the prosthesis can be expected to function for 10 years in at least 85% or more of the patients.

While it is possible to replace a joint replacement with another joint replacement, that is, to do a revision operation, this is more tedious and dangerous than a primary intervention. Much of the bone stock required to implant the prosthesis has thinned or is gone altogether. Chances of excessive blood loss (due to longer operating time and the previous disturbance of the tissue), infection, and postoperative problems are all greater with revision operations. Overall, the final results of revision operations, while still good, are not as good as those following the primary operation. Joint replacements are most indicated in those patients in whom a revision should not be necessary.

For all the above reasons, total joint operations tend to be limited to patients who are over the age of 60, who are willing to accept the limitations of no heavy work and no athletic activity, who are at or near ideal body weight and weigh, preferably, less than 200 pounds, and who are willing to accept the risks of the operation. The procedure can be considered for younger patients who have some built-in physical restraint (*e.g.,* generalized arthritis involving most of the joints of the body, severe cardiopulmonary disease, or leukemia) which will not permit them normal activity even after total joint replacement. These indications are virtually the same for both hip and knee replacement.

The chances of success with a joint replacement (in the immediate postoperative period) with satisfactory range of motion and virtually pain-free function are better than 95%. The risks are those associated with any operation (from anesthesia in an older age group, postoperative phlebitis, pulmonary embolus, urinary tract infection, etc.). However, the most dangerous risk with joint replacement is that of infection in the operative wound. As with any foreign body, if an implant becomes infected, the implant almost always must be removed. Until recently it was taught that any infection of a joint replacement required complete removal of the prosthesis, and that no prosthesis could ever be implanted in its place. Some successful reimplantations of prostheses into infected beds have been accomplished but, in most cases, a significant, deep postoperative infection implies failure.

Chapter 8

Pain in the Back and Leg

Eric L. Radin and Jamshid Tehranzadeh

A substantial industry has developed to provide treatment for patients with low back pain. Osteopaths, chiropractors, physical therapists, trainers, druggists, and a number of self-styled "experts" offer cures and advice. There is a whole literature of self-help programs available from any library or bookstore. The reason for this is that organized medicine's approach to low back pain patients is inadequate. The degree of success in treating patients with pain in the back radiating to the leg has been so low that most practitioners are depressed at the presentation of these patients, and some orthopaedic surgeons simply refuse to treat low back pain. Part of the trouble is that low back pain is a common symptom with multiple causes, and treating physicians are frequently schooled to recognize only one set of causes, neurologic. A complicating factor is that the psychic potentiation of chronic low back pain is an effective and socially acceptable conversion syndrome.

An understanding of the pathophysiology of low back and leg pain and the ability to recognize psychic potentiation when it presents itself should permit effective treatment of the majority of patients. This chapter will discuss the causes of low back and leg pain within this context.

Causes of Back Pain

Pulled Muscle

The most common cause of low back pain is back strain resulting from a pulled muscle. Muscles tear when they are accidentally stretched during contraction. This occurs most frequently when a person is lifting a heavy object and the object falls or the person's position is abruptly and unexpectedly changed. The back is then forced into a new position while the muscles used to stabilize the spine are contracted. The sudden change causes these muscles to stretch and tear (Fig. 8-1). This back strain is associated with the acute onset of pain and diffuse low back tenderness with muscle spasm.

Ninety-five percent of acute low back pain is from pulled muscles. Torn muscles in continuity heal within 6 weeks, even without treatment. Ligamentous tears (sprains) are rare in the spine and are usually the result of an automobile accident or a fall from a great height. Ruptured intervertebral discs, the diagnosis all physicians try to make, probably represent the cause in less than 5% of patients with acute low back pain.

Ruptured Intervertebral Disc, Spondylosis, and Sciatica

Pathology in the back is frequently perceived by a patient as pain in the back, leg, or both. The lower extremities and the lumbar and lumbosacral spines are innervated by the same spinal nerve roots, L4–S1. Irritation of these nerve roots will be sensed in their dermatomic distribution; that is, pain in the back will radiate to the leg. This is commonly referred to as "sciatica" and is best classified as either neurogenic in origin (true sciatica) or mechanical in origin (apparent or referred sciatica). However, the pain may also have other causes, including vascular abnormalities (as from a ruptured abdominal aortic aneurysm), intrapelvic or retroperitoneal lesions, neoplasms (especially metastasis or myeloma in older patients), inflammatory arthritis affecting the spine (such as rheumatoid arthritis or ankylosing spondylosis), and osteoporotic fractures. Paget's disease can also cause back and leg pain.

Renal stones, prostatitis, retrocecal appendicitis, and other intrapelvic lesions can occasionally present themselves as low back pain, as can hip disease. The former can be distinguished from lumbosacral pathology by history and physical examination, the latter by reproducing the symptoms by hip motions while the back is still. Since hip flexion can be accompanied by lumbosacral motion, the physician should examine hip rotation with the hip extended.

True sciatica is pain caused by direct pressure on the lower lumbar or sacral roots which form or constitute the sciatic nerve. It can be caused by a neurapraxia (pressure on a nerve) anywhere along the

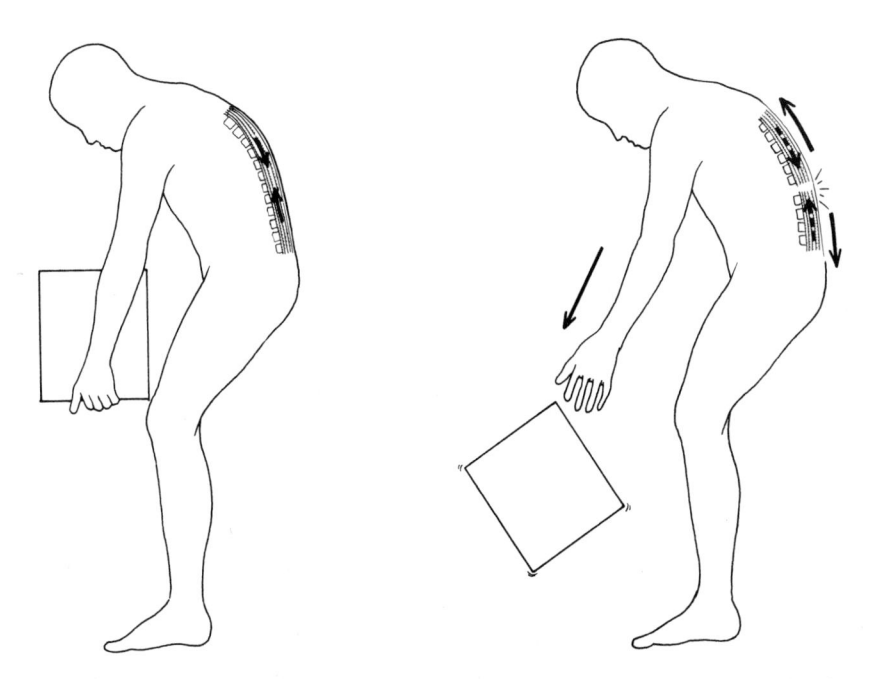

Figure 8-1. The paraspinal muscles can be torn if they are contracted and stretched at the same time, as occurs when suddenly reaching for a heavy load that has been dropped.

nerve. Most commonly, however, it will be caused by posterior extrusion of intervertebral disc material pressing on a spinal root as it emerges from the cauda equina, passes over the posterior part of the intervertebral disc, and continues through the bony intervertebral foramen. Posterior disc rupture is most common at L5–S1 because of the oblique angulation of that interspace (Fig. 8-2). The other interspaces, for the most part, are horizontal. Pressure on a lumbar or upper sacral nerve root can be caused by a rupture of the annulus fibrosus with extrusion of a fragment of disc material. The fragment may break off and lodge in the intervertebral foramen. A posteriorly bulging annulus fibrosus is common, is related to age, and does not cause nerve root pressure in an otherwise normal spine (Fig. 8-3).

The history given by a patient with an acute ruptured disc is generally one of acute onset, usually related to an episode of combined forward flexion and twisting of the lumbosacral spine. One does not have to be lifting something heavy to rupture an annulus fibrosus and extrude disc material; however, patients frequently are engaged in

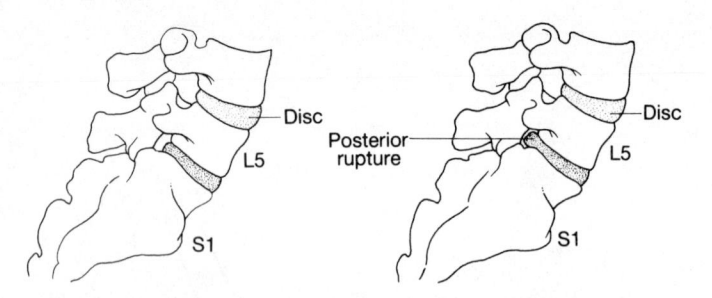

Figure 8-2. The L5–S1 interspace has an oblique orientation, so there tends to be a forward slipping of L5 on S1 when we stand. As a result, the L5–S1 disc is subjected to high stress and posterior rupture.

heavy lifting when they are injured. It has been shown experimentally that a combination of flexion and axial rotation puts the highest pressure across the disc, and that this combination of motions is necessary to tear the annulus fibrosus. The pain from a ruptured disc is usually constant, but can be relieved by positions that take the pressure off the posterior intervertebral disc area, such as flexion of the spine.

Patients with acute ruptured intervertebral disc are not comfortable sitting but are frequently comfortable lying, especially with the knees bent. The highest pressures across the intervertebral disc are created by sitting, as opposed to standing or lying. The major load across all joints is created by the muscular contraction crossing those joints, which is necessary to stabilize them. For the spine, paravertebral muscular contraction is essential to maintain a seated posture. Paralyzed

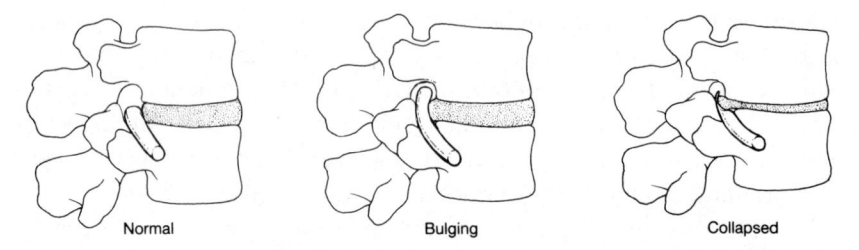

Figure 8-3. The disc impingement from a collapsed interspace on the intervertebral foramen through which the nerve root passes significantly narrows the foramen. Bulging discs without actual rupture should not be considered pathological.

people cannot sit independently. When standing, a person positions the center of gravity over the feet, contracts the abdominal muscles, and, hence, requires less stabilization from the muscles of the spine. Lying requires no extrinsic spinal stabilization and totally relaxes the paraspinal muscles. Bending the knees functionally shortens the sciatic nerves and flexes the lumbosacral junction, opening it up posteriorly, further reducing the pressure on the nerve roots. This explains why such patients tend to want to flex their knees in bed.

On physical examination, there may be localized tenderness over the involved intervertebral space, muscle spasm, limitation of back motion, and signs of neurapraxia (*i.e.,* motor, sensory, and reflex deficits). The distribution of pain is not reliably pathognomonic for a ruptured disc. Myelography will usually demonstrate an extradural filling defect.

An inflammatory response generally accompanies a ruptured intervertebral disc, and this inflammatory response is capable, over several weeks, of digesting away the herniated nucleus pulposus material. Ninety-five percent of patients with acute ruptured intervertebral discs with neurologic signs will improve with conservative measures in 6 to 12 weeks. The indications for surgery are failure to improve on bed rest, documented increase in the degree of neurologic involvement, or bladder control involvement. Removal of extruding disc material should then be carried out.

Pain of mechanical origin in the low back arises most commonly from L5–S1 due to degenerative changes of the intervertebral facets. This spinal segment is the one most commonly involved in a deteriorative process because of the shear forces on it due to its obliquity. Since the intervertebral joints are innervated by the spinal root that passes next to them, the L5–S1 intervertebral facets are innervated by the L5 nerve root. Pain here will be read by pain centers in the brain as a pain coming from the back and the L5 distribution of the leg. It will simulate sciatica. Apparent sciatica is pain in the sciatic distribution from causes other than neurapraxia. It is referred pain. Joint pain is commonly referred to more distal portions of the body (*e.g.,* pain from the hip is frequently experienced in the thigh or knee).

The ligaments and the L5–S1 intervertebral facet joints keep the L5 vertebral body from slipping forward on S1. Bony abnormalities at this level are common, afflicting about 15% of the population, and may predispose affected individuals to wear and tear of the facets. Osteoarthrosis of the L5–S1 intervertebral joints, manifested by narrowing of

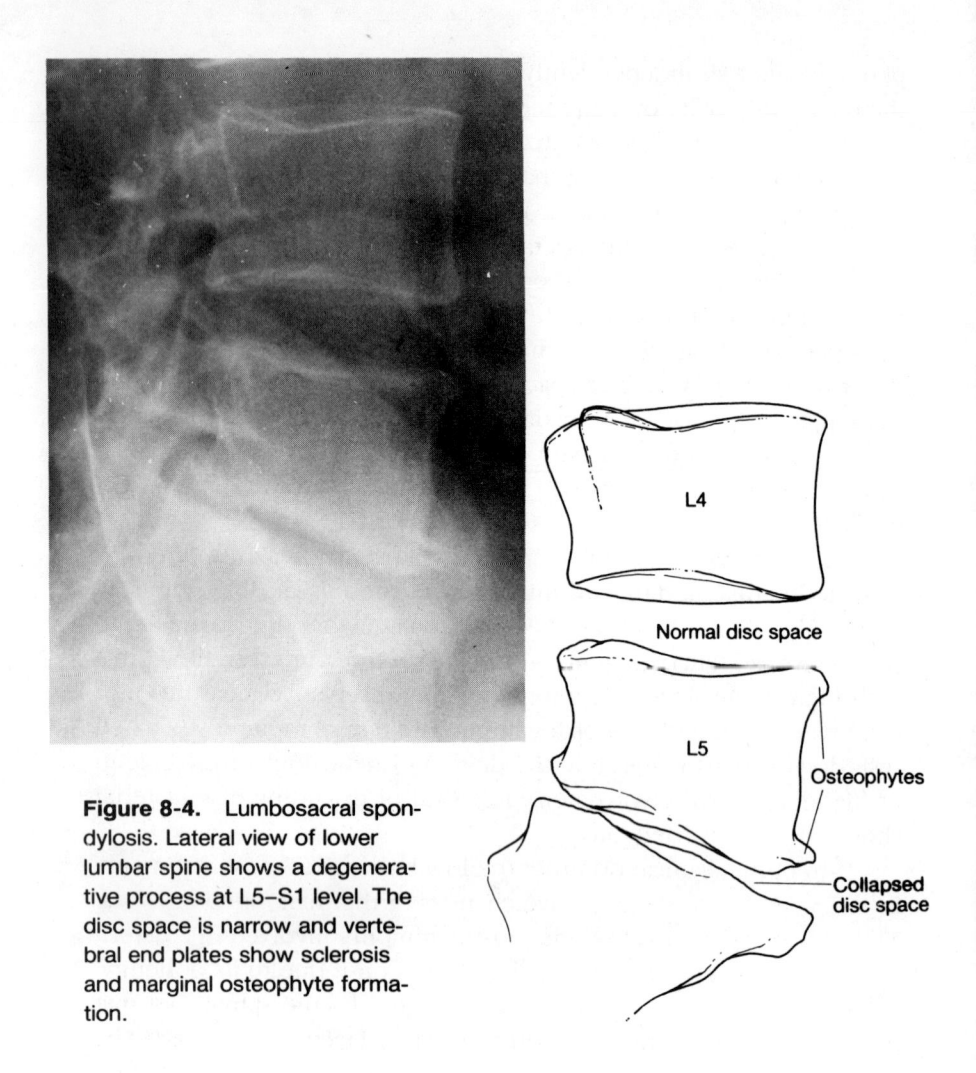

Figure 8-4. Lumbosacral spondylosis. Lateral view of lower lumbar spine shows a degenerative process at L5–S1 level. The disc space is narrow and vertebral end plates show sclerosis and marginal osteophyte formation.

the joint space, sclerosis, and hypertrophic change at the joints, is called *spondylosis* (Fig. 8-4).

Disc loss with intervertebral body interspace narrowing inevitably leads to osteoarthrotic changes. The intervertebral joint must be thought of as the combination of the intervertebral disc and the intervertebral facet joints. One part of this structure cannot be altered or damaged without affecting the other. Because the facets are congruous in fit when there is a disc, they will no longer fit when the disc space is collapsed. This phenomenon makes the advantages of conservative treatment for patients with ruptured discs clear; surgical "clean-out" of the vertebral interspace will further distort an already narrowed disc space and cause greater incongruity in the way the facet joints fit together. The same phenomenon suggests that interbody fusions, which maintain the disc space after disc excision, may have better long-term success than procedures that empty the disc space and allow it to collapse. Spondylosis, then, is manifested on x-ray film by disc-space narrowing as well as by facet joint deterioration and bony proliferation.

The treating physician cannot count on being able to differentiate true sciatica from sciatica of spondylitic origin by the character and distribution of the pain. Generally, the pain of spondylosis at L5–S1 is characteristically aggravated by sitting or standing for prolonged periods of time and relieved by lying down for a few minutes, but this may not always be true. The important distinctions can be made on physical examination. Although both ruptured intervertebral discs and spondylosis will give localized tenderness at L5–S1 (or the involved interspace) and painful limitation of motion of the spinal segments involved, the presence or absence of neurologic signs (*i.e.,* motor, sensory, or reflex deficits) is the only reliable differentiating diagnostic indication.

Pain in the back on straight leg raising, unfortunately, is not pathognomonic of a ruptured intervertebral disc, as it can arise from any retroperitoneal or intrapelvic pathology, including retrocecal appendicitis. Since straight leg raising involves flexion of the hip as well as the lumbosacral junctions, inflammation of either hip or lumbosacral joint will cause pain or limitation of straight leg raising. Tenderness of the sciatic or perineal nerve is a helpful sign, as is pain in the sciatic distribution of the painful side on contralateral straight leg raising. This pain is thought to be caused by fixation or trapping of a nerve root in the spinal column or foramen by an extruded disc fragment. Pulling on the opposite root will pull on the involved root as well. In some patients with disc herniation, there is pain in the leg on straight leg raising, which is relieved by bending the knee and aggravated by dorsiflexing the ankle, again the result of irritability of the roots of the sciatic nerve (Lasègue's sign). Unfortunately, a number of the patients who seemed to develop this sign had the pain suggested to them during prior examinations. For this reason, straight leg raising has not proved to be as reliable as other signs.

Myelography is of limited usefulness in distinguishing spondylosis from acute ruptured intervertebral discs. Although a myelogram may show an extradural defect in a symptomatic individual, the defect may

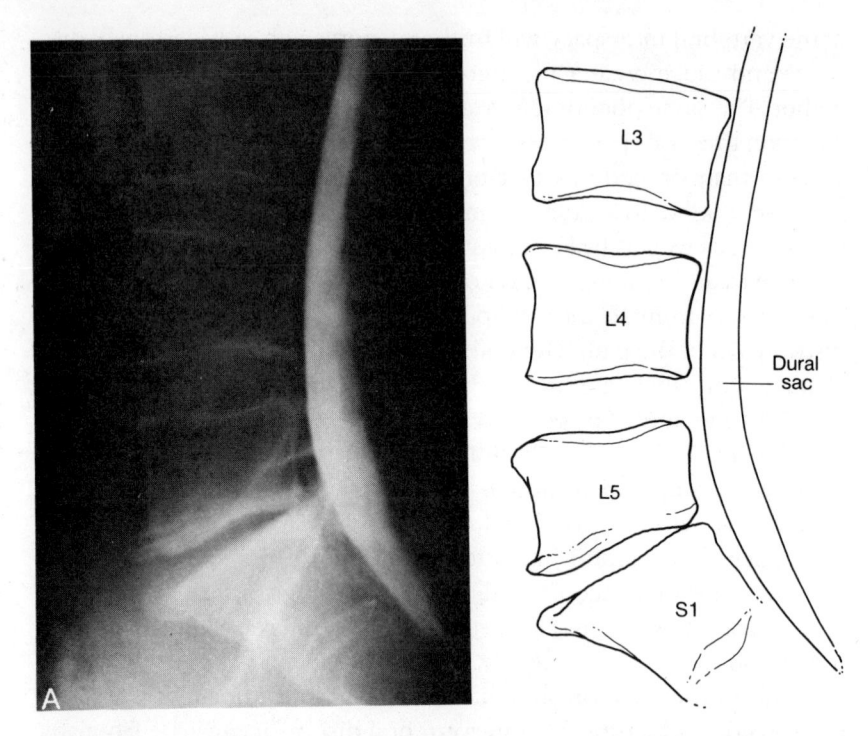

Figure 8-5. *A:* Normal metrizamide myelogram (lateral view). Note the smooth margins of the contrast-filled dural sac. The L5–S1 disc space is collapsed, but there is no evidence of disc rupture at this time.

represent scarring from an old disc rupture that is no longer symptomatic (Fig. 8-5 *A, B*). The myelogram cannot distinguish between scar and disc material; thus, it cannot distinguish between symptomatic and asymptomatic defects and is useful only when considered in context with the history and physical findings. Myelograms are helpful, however, in diagnosing other intraspinal pathology, such as tumors or congenital abnormalities. Computed tomography (CT scan) has improved the accuracy of myelograms because it frequently allows one to distinguish between scar and disc material. It will also demonstrate hypertrophied bony or ligamentous encroachment on the spinal canal (Fig. 8-6 *A, B*).

It has been found that the enzyme chymopapain will cause disc shrinkage if directly injected. Although there are some serious, potential side-effects, these injections have successfully relieved disc herniation symptoms in about 50% to 70% of appropriate cases. Enzymatic

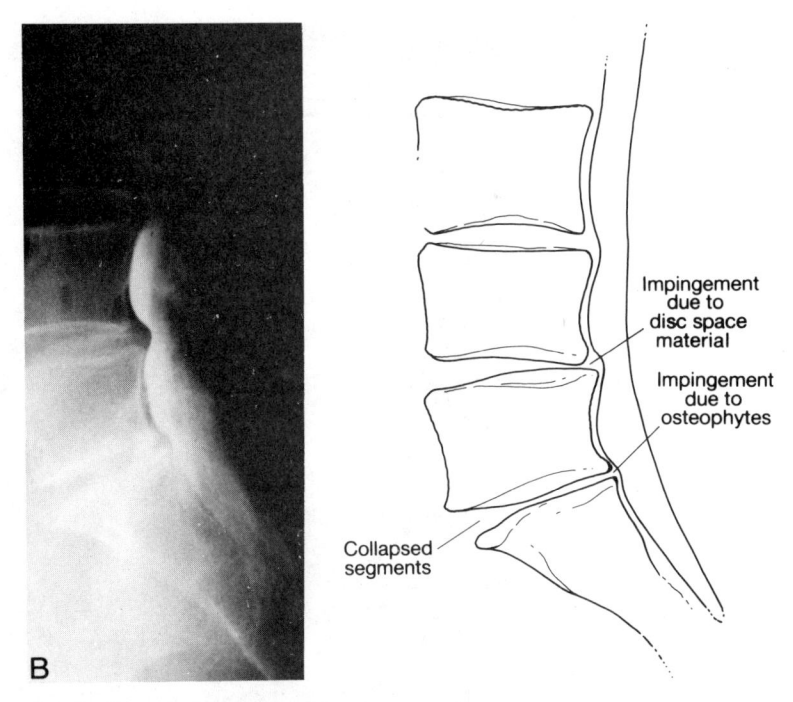

Figure 8-5. *B:* Metrizamide myelogram (lateral view) showing multiple impingements on the contrast-filled dural sac due to ruptured disc and osteophyte formation.

injection of intervertebral discs seems to lead to the same disc space narrowing and spondylosis as does surgical "clean-out." Chymopapain appears to have the same long-term complication of eventual spondylosis as does surgical disc excision.

Spinal fluid analysis can be helpful in ruling out tumors associated with very high spinal fluid proteins, interspinal infections, or inflammatory conditions.

Failure to understand that most ruptured intervertebral discs will heal with scar and to appreciate the fact that myelograms are not diagnostic of acute ruptured discs, that surgery itself can lead to scarring and neurapraxia, and that disc loss will lead to spondylosis has helped to give disc surgery the poor reputation it currently enjoys. Studies have shown that only 50% of patients stay improved after surgery for acute ruptured disc. In a randomly selected series of cases, patients do just as well without surgery.

122 Adult Orthopaedic Problems

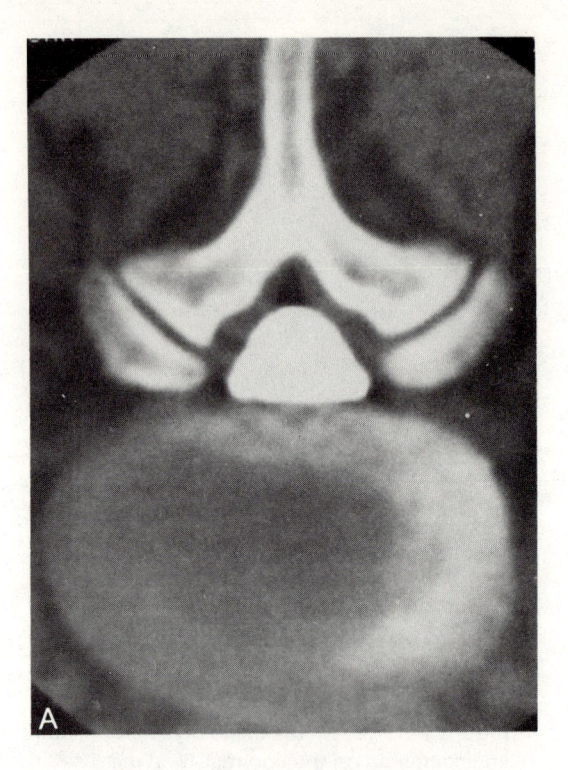

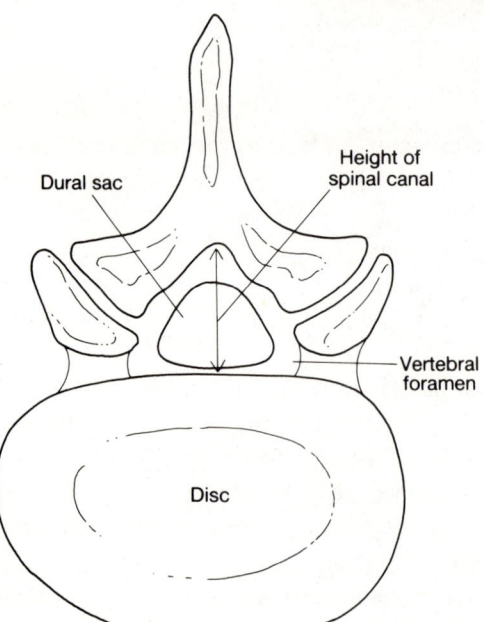

Figure 8-6. *A:* Axial tomography of a normal lumbar intervertebral space.

Pain in the Back and Leg   123

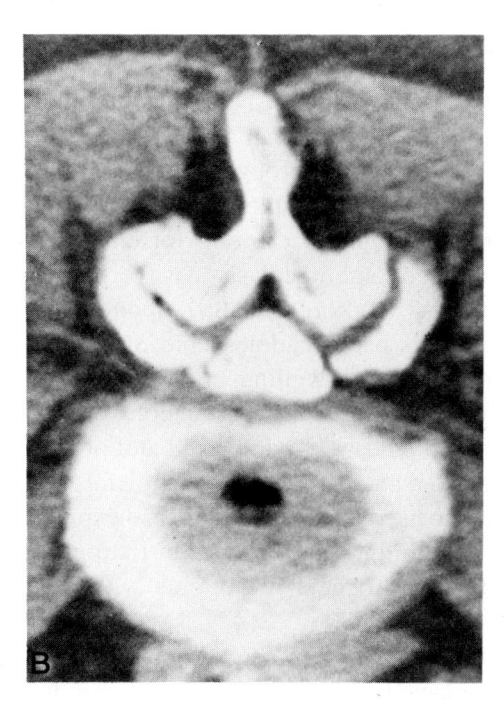

Figure 8-6. *B:* Axial tomography of a lumbar spine of a patient with spondylosis and old disc herniation. There are hypertrophic changes, narrowing, and deformity of intervertebral facet joints. The lateral neural foramens and spinal canal are narrowed. The bony hypertrophy has narrowed the spinal canal encroaching on and squeezing the cauda equina, creating a spinal stenosis.

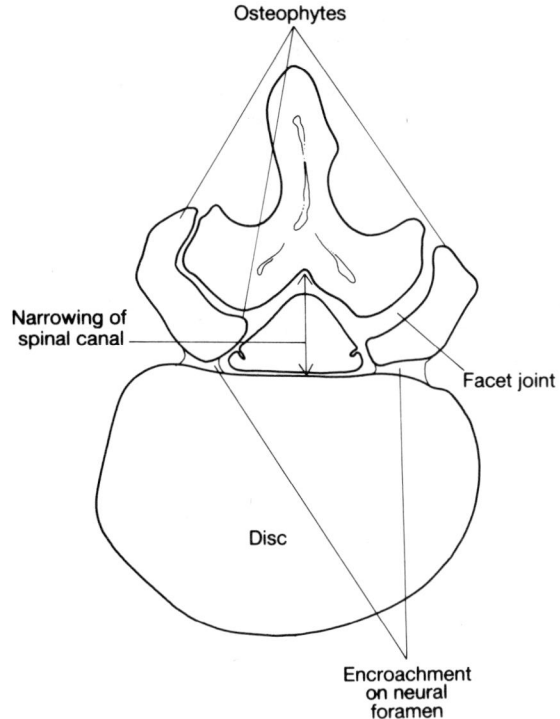

Spondylolysis and Spondylolisthesis

Instability of the lumbosacral junction can also be painful and is either caused by a congenital bony insufficiency or is an abnormality of acquired damage, commonly a stress fracture through the pars interarticularis that causes the facet joints to be unstable. In the absence of an intact pars, the lower vertebral segment can slip forward (Fig. 8-7). The bony inadequacy is called "spondylolysis" (if there is no slip forward) or "spondylolisthesis" (if there is a slip). Spondylolisthesis is the major cause of low back pain in adolescents. Since pain results mainly from inflammation and local swelling, or from increased interosseous venous pressure, there is not always a correlation between bony change and pain. Radiographic changes can be old and of long standing, and may be unrelated to a patient's current complaint. The relationship between pain and increased venous pressure also explains why pain exacerbation with coughing, sneezing, and straining is not limited to true sciatica but also occurs in patients with joint involvement.

Treatment for spondylosis, spondylolysis, or spondylolisthesis involves relieving the muscle spasm and joint inflammation, and splinting the abdominal muscles with a corset or girdle. This treatment increases the hydrostatic intra-abdominal pressure, providing anterior support for the lumbar spine, and helps to tighten the oblique abdominal lumbodorsal fascia, which further supports the bones. Splinting with something rigid, such as plaster or fiberglass body jackets or metal braces, may be indicated if a corset is inadequate. Spondylosis is the second-most-common cause of low back pain and occurs particularly in older age groups. Spondylolisthesis can be activity-related and is common in football linemen and gymnasts, who subject their lumbosacral junctions to considerable shearing impacts. Spinal fusion may be indicated for persistence of severe symptomatic joint instability.

Spinal Stenosis

Spondylosis with its associated proliferation of bony lips and spurs can itself cause impingement on the cauda equina within the spinal canal (see Fig. 8-6*B*). This process is very insidious in onset. Its primary symptoms are low back pain and radiating leg pain that occur, characteristically, after walking. This *spinal claudication,* like arterial claudication, resolves within a minute or two if the patient stops walk-

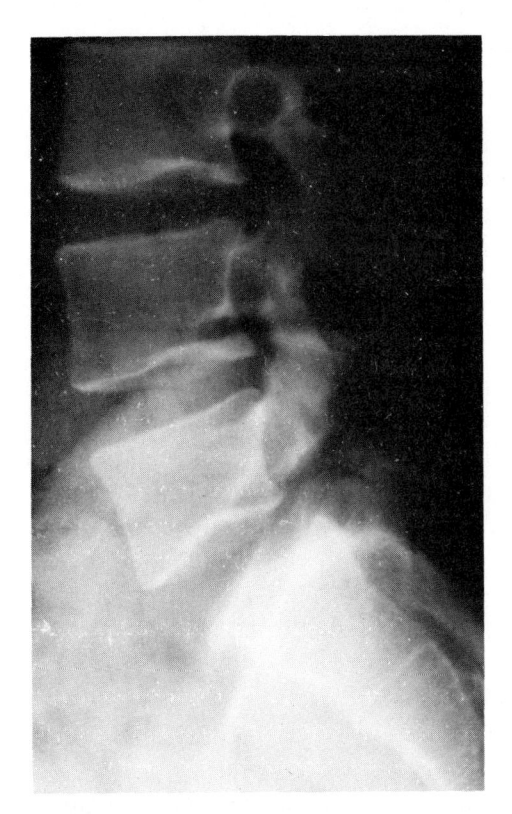

Figure 8-7. Bony defect of posterior spinal elements allows the L5 vertebral body to slip forward on S1 creating a spondylolisthesis.

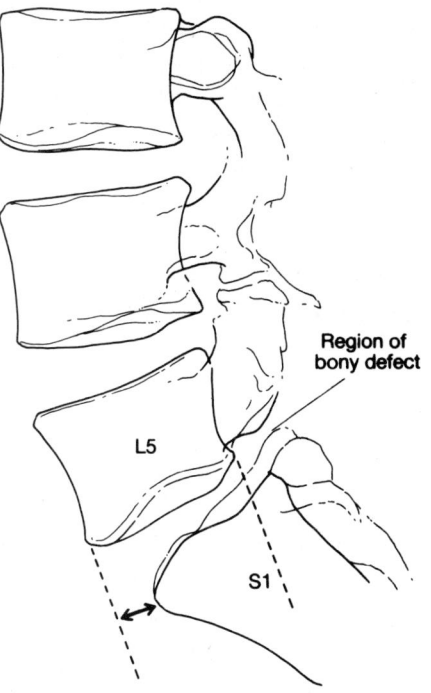

ing. Frequently, flexing the lumbosacral spine as in a squatting position also helps to relieve the discomfort, as does sitting. The pain occurs after the individual has walked certain distances and is severe enough to cause the patient to stop the activity. The symptoms are quite reproducible; as time passes the distance walked before symptoms occur becomes shorter and shorter.

Treatment involves increasing the size of the spinal canal, usually by laminectomy. The diagnosis is made from the characteristic history and CT scan appearance. There are usually no physical findings other than those associated with spondylosis. This is not neurologic loss. It is presumed that in gait there is some motion of the cauda equina and that when this occurs in a tight place, local swelling will occur. Others feel that the nutrient vessels to the spinal cord can be compressed over bony ridges and that "spinal claudication" has the same physiology as arterial claudication. Both factors may actually play a role in causing this condition.

Psychological Factors

The psychic potentiation of low back symptoms beyond their "physiologic life" is common and complicates treatment. The reasons for potentiation, which is frequently unconscious, are usually social or economic gain. If the pain is the result of an accident that occurred at work or is covered by insurance the economic benefit is obvious. The social benefit may not be so clear. Individuals with acute low back pain are excused from their work and domestic duties; since this happens without loss of face or feelings of inadequacy, it may be extremely gratifying psychologically. The Minnesota Multiphasic Personality Inventory (MMPI) has been a useful indicator in spotting such reactions. Many of these patients, however, object to psychiatric help.

Management of Acute Muscle Strains of the Back

The management of back pain is primarily dependent upon the presence or absence of objective signs localized to a particular interspace. Patients with objective neurologic signs should almost always be treated with some degree of enforced recumbency for a specified period of time. The overwhelming majority of patients with low back pain have muscle strains, though, and bed rest is not necessarily indicated. The time-tested treatment of muscle strains of the back consists of the following recommendations:

1. Painful activities should be limited. This may or may not mean bed rest.
2. The patient should sleep or rest on a comfortable bed. A bed board may help.
3. Some form of heat should be applied to the back. Deep heat provides an additional degree of comfort but is not mandatory.
4. Some form of non-narcotic analgesic should be used. Aspirin, 600 to 900 mg four times a day, is by far the simplest and most effective. The patient should be cautioned to take the aspirin with a full glass of water or at mealtime, and to discontinue use if tinnitus or gastric irritation arises.
5. The patient should carry with him a commercially available semirigid back-support pad measuring 12" × 16" (30 × 40 cm). These are particularly effective for patients who complain of backache while driving. Sometimes a magazine, inserted between the seat and the back, can splint the back. A molded bucket seat, available from various sources, can help.
6. A canvas type of lumbosacral support corset might be useful to some patients as a temporary measure, particularly those with weak or stretched abdominal muscles.
7. Exercises should be undertaken to strengthen the abdominal and back muscles after the acute pain has subsided. These should not be prescribed during the acute phase of backache and are only indicated for patients who are prone to backache.

Part Four

Pediatric Orthopaedic Problems

Chapter 9

Congenital and Developmental Conditions

Eric T. Jones

We depend upon growth to develop normal bones and joints. Growth can, however, produce deformity, as in cerebral palsy, where spastic and unbalanced muscle forces gradually deform bones and joints that were normal at birth. Conversely, with proper management, a child born with metatarsus adductus, clubfoot, or congenital dislocation of the hip has the potential, with growth, to develop a near-normal foot or hip if the deformity is corrected early in the child's development. Soft-tissue contractures, such as a tight heel cord, will, if left uncorrected, cause the bones to grow in this abnormal position, changing a soft-tissue deformity into a bony one. Thus, correction of deformities in the growing child should be carried out as soon as possible.

Bone Formation and Growth

Embryonic bone forms either through *intramembranous* or *endochondral ossification*. In the former, mesenchymal cells proliferate to form membranes primarily in the region in which flat bones will be fabricated. Ossification continues in the membrane, and a sheet of bone covered by mesenchymal cells is formed. The surface cells become the periosteum. The primary bone is remodeled, and with the ingrowth of blood vessels a medullary space is formed.

Endochondral ossification is bony replacement of a cartilage model and is the mode of formation of long bones (Fig. 9-1). Early in gestation mesenchymal cells aggregate to form models of the future long bones.

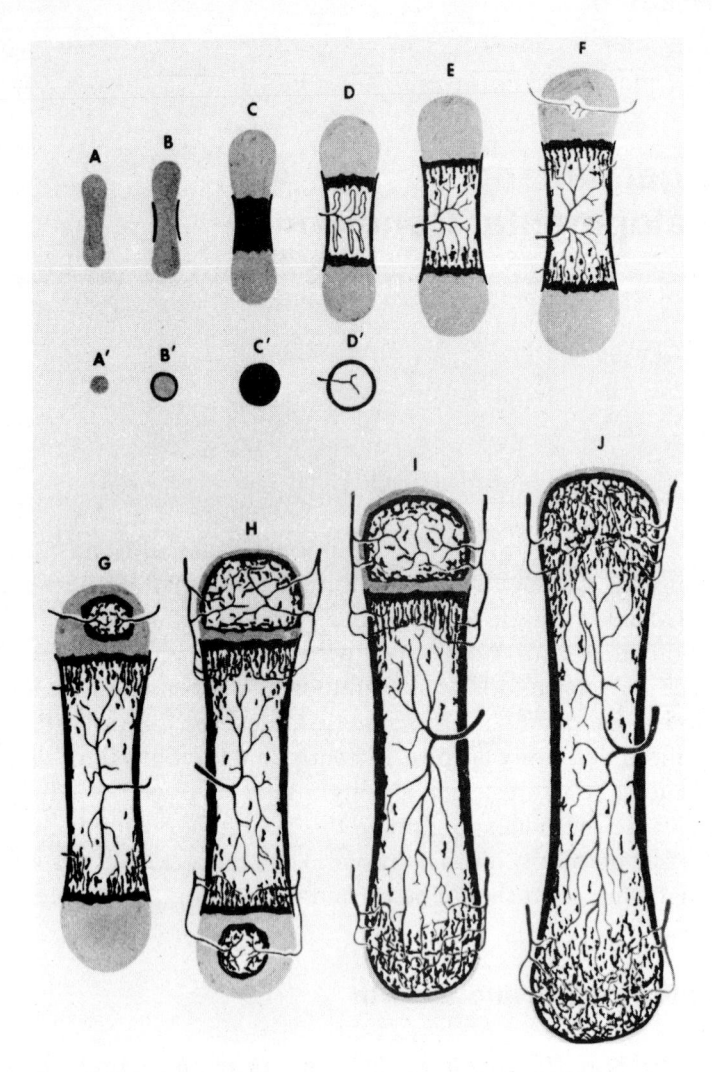

Figure 9-1. Diagrammatic development of a typical long bone (longitudinal sections A through J and cross sections A', B', C', D' through the centers of A, B, C, and D). *A:* cartilage model. *B:* periosteal bone appears before any calcification of cartilage. *C:* cartilage begins to calcify. *D:* vascular mesenchyma enters the calcified cartilage matrix and divides it into two zones of ossification (*E*). *F:* blood vessels and mesenchyma enter the upper epiphyseal cartilage and the epiphyseal ossification center develops in it (*G*). *H:* a similar ossification center develops in the lower epiphyseal cartilage. As the bone ceases to grow in length, the lower epiphyseal plate disappears first (*I*) followed

A cartilage model develops and the peripheral cells organize into a perichondrium. The cartilage cells enlarge and degenerate, and the matrix surrounding them calcifies. The enveloping perichondrium of the region converts to a periosteum and deposits a layer of compact bone peripherally, through a process of intramembranous ossification. As these events occur, a vascular bud enters the ossification center, bringing with it new mesenchymal cells that will modulate into bone-forming cells. This primary center of ossification, located in the diaphysis, extends toward both metaphyseal regions. The terminal ends of the cartilage model continue to grow in length by cartilage cell proliferation.

Long-bone growth continues in this manner until after birth, when secondary ossification centers (epiphyses) develop. Vessels grow into the cartilaginous ends of the bone and form secondary centers of ossification. In later postnatal development, the mass of cartilage cells found between the epiphyseal and diaphyseal bone thins to become the epiphyseal plate, which continues as the principal contributor to longitudinal growth of long bones until maturation is reached (Fig. 9-2).

There are many factors known to function in the development, physiology, and rate of growth of the epiphyseal plate. Growth hormone is a constant factor stimulating the growth plate. Other known factors affecting growth include individual genetic makeup, nutrition, and adrenal and gonadal androgens and estrogens. They influence both the rate of bone growth and the time of appearance of the secondary ossification centers.

The girth of the long bone is provided by the inner layer of the periosteum. Successive surfaces of compact bone are added to the exterior, while remodeling by resorption of the interior (endosteal) surface takes place (Fig. 9-3).

The typical long bone usually develops from one diaphyseal and two epiphyseal ossification centers. Longitudinal growth occurs by new endochondral bone formation "pushing" the epiphyses away from the

---

by the upper epiphyseal plate (*J*). The marrow cavity then becomes continuous throughout the length of the bone and the blood vessels of the diaphysis, metaphysis, and epiphyses intercommunicate. (Bloom W, Fawcett DW: Textbook of Histology, p 247. Philadelphia, WB Saunders, 1968)

134 Pediatric Orthopaedic Problems

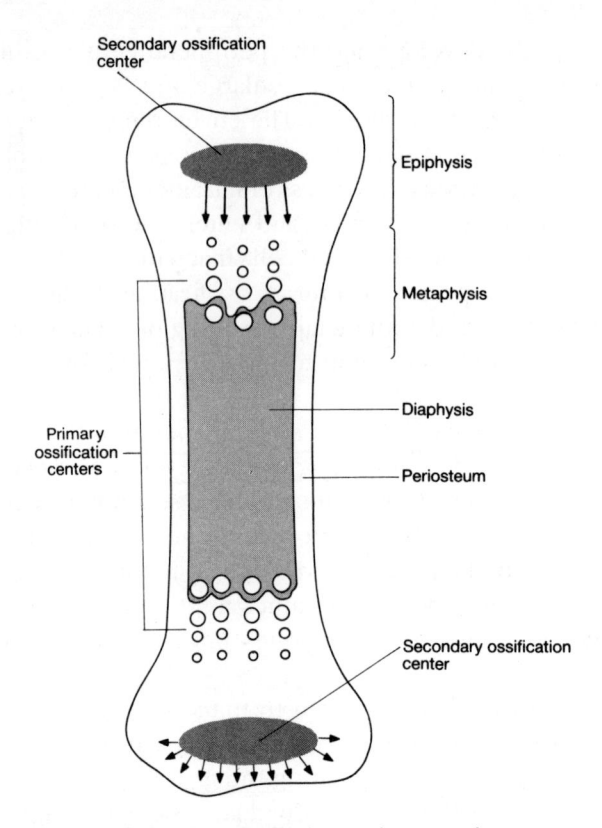

Figure 9-2. Longitudinal growth occurs by new endochondral bone formation, "pushing" the epiphysis away from the metaphysis as illustrated at the upper epiphysis. Articular ends grow by endochondral new-bone formation from the secondary ossification center.

metaphysis (see Fig. 9-2). Circumferential growth is intramembranous from the diaphyseal periosteum. The epiphyses (articulating ends) grow from endochondral ossification as though the secondary ossification center is a spherical metaphysis enlarging in all directions. The smaller long bones of the hands and feet have one diaphyseal and one epiphyseal ossification center, while the small bones (carpals and tarsals) ossify from one center.

The longitudinal growth rate of extremities is at its greatest just after birth. Thus a growth-plate injury or infection can cause a significant

Congenital and Developmental Conditions **135**

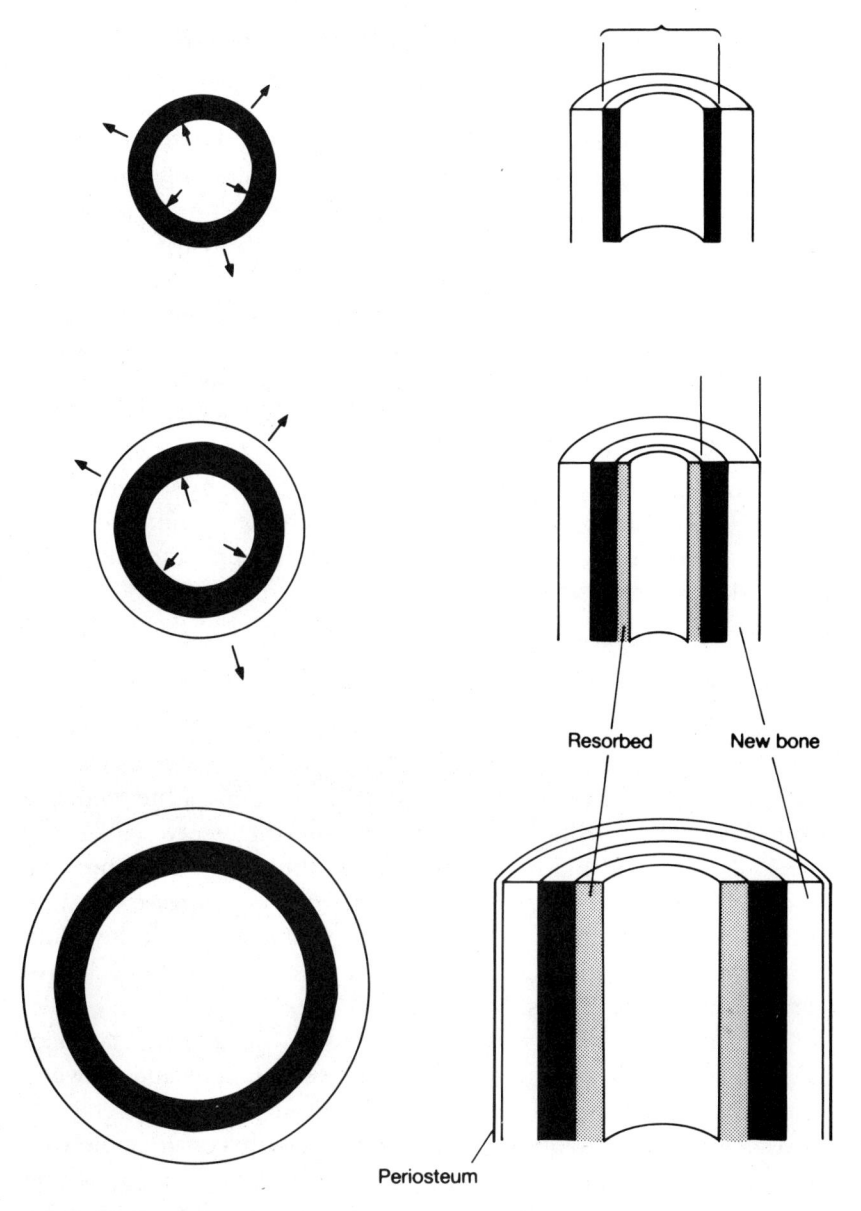

Figure 9-3. Circumferential growth of the shaft is intramembranous bone formation from the diaphyseal periosteum. It is associated with endosteal resorption.

limb-length or angular discrepancy when the insult is to a young, growing child.

The neonatal period provides a unique opportunity for those involved in the management of skeletal deformity. Although supported by scant experimental documentation, there is evidence of a temporary ligamentous laxity in the neonate, secondary to maternal hormones such as relaxin and estrogens. This short period of hyperelasticity, coupled with the rapid growth of the neonate, can facilitate correction of deformity. If the deforming forces are appropriately managed, the adaptive pathological changes can be reversed, and in many cases avoided altogether. For example, early stretching exercises can, in some cases, correct a newborn's inward turning (adducted) forefeet within several months. If left unstretched, the deformity will persist and become a fixed bony abnormality, uncorrectable by stretching exercises. If a condition such as a congenitally dislocated hip is allowed to persist, the problem becomes more complex and the treatment required more extensive.

Normal Infant Development

The axial skeleton changes shape with growth. A newborn's entire spine is concave anteriorly; in the first three months of life, with the acquisition of head control, cervical lordosis (the reserve curve) appears (Fig. 9-4). Similarly, lumbar lordosis begins with sitting. The axial skeleton does not contribute as much to overall increase in height in childhood as do the lower extremities. Compared with the adult, the neonate has a relatively large head and long spine, with disproportionately shorter limbs.

In evaluating infants with orthopaedic problems, it is important to consider the physiologic variations between infants and between infants and older children or adults. Variations in uterine and fetal size and differences in intrauterine activity may result in considerable variation among newborns in both the active and passive range of motion of joints. A newborn may lack as much as 30° of active and passive elbow extension, while the range of motion in other upper-extremity joints may approximate that of an adult. In the newborn, hips and knees are usually held flexed, and the tibiae are bowed and are usually internally rotated. Hip flexion contracture of 50° to 120° may be present. The knees may lack up to 30° of full extension (there should be

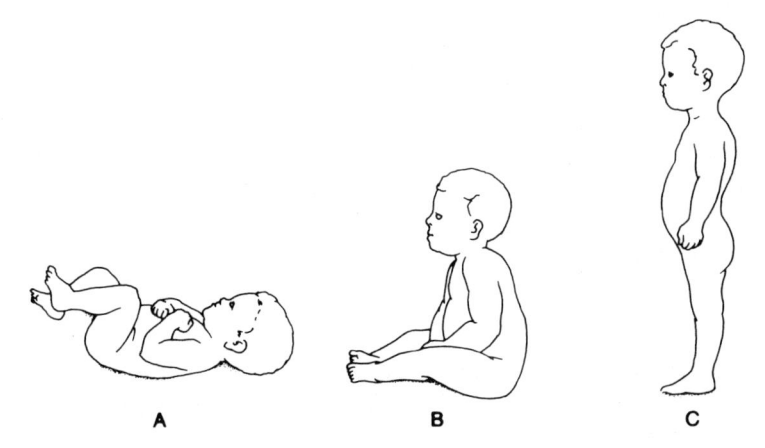

Figure 9-4. In the newborn the spine is anteriorly concave (*A*). With head control the child gains cervical lordosis (*B*), and with standing gains lumbar lordosis (*C*). (After Tachdjian MO: Pediatric Orthopedics, vol 2, p 1140. Philadelphia, WB Saunders, 1972)

full flexion). The feet and ankles may be found in many interesting positions, most of which are probably related to intrauterine molding. Ankle dorsiflexion of 60°, compared with plantar flexion of neutral to 30°, can be normal in a newborn, making the foot appear to be bent forward on the tibia. These positions are rapidly corrected spontaneously.

Rotational Variation

As the extremities grow longitudinally, they also change rotationally and angularly, and important physiologic variations occur. Most of the lower-extremity rotational "problems" seen in infants represent either side of the normal physiologic variation at each stage of growth and development. These rotational variations are commonly present in the first two years of life, and their source may be at one level or at several levels of the lower extremities. In infancy, the most common conditions causing rotational variation are medial tibial torsion, external rotatory contracture of the hip, and metatarsus adductus.

All children with a rotational variation should be examined to rule out the possibility of a pathologic condition such as cerebral palsy, myelodysplasia, diastematomyelia (congenital abnormality of the

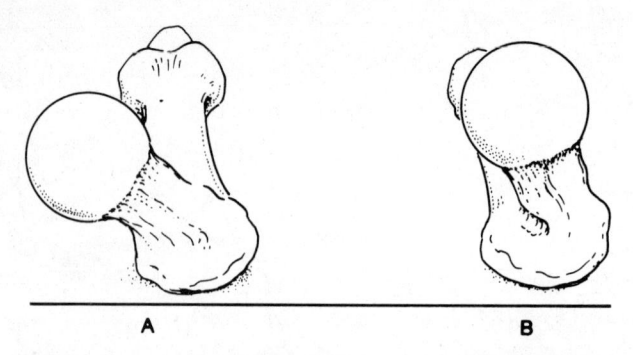

Figure 9-5. *A:* Infantile degree of femoral neck anteversion, as viewed from the top. *B:* more normal (adult degree) of femoral anteversion. If the infantile degree of anteversion persists, the individual's whole leg will be rotated inward in compensation.

spinal canal), or a subtle neurologic problem. The child who has asymmetrical findings or a history of a progressive deformity is particularly suspect, since these are not characteristic of the usual rotational problem. The child must be cooperative for an adequate evaluation to be made. A stepwise examination of the nonwalking child with a rotational variant should include examination for foot deformity and for tibial or femoral rotation or bowing, and evaluation of the range of motion of the ankle, knee, and hip. The examination isolates sequentially the foot, the tibia, and the femur, and permits assessment of their role in the rotational problem. The natural history of these conditions usually favors improvement with time. Most require only conservative treatment, such as stretching and night splints; surgical intervention is rarely necessary.

Femoral Anteversion. Internal femoral torsion is an abnormal relationship of the femoral shaft to the head and neck of the femur. Normally the head and neck of the femur are directed forward (anteverted) relative to the femoral shaft (Fig. 9-5). If the degree of infantile anteversion persists, the whole leg will be rotated inward; the child will toe in and there will be a limitation of external rotation of the hip in extension. Interestingly, a compensating external rotation of the tibial shaft frequently develops with growth as the child tries to get his feet to point forward. External hip rotation is limited because the posterior neck, now situated very far backwards, and the greater trochanter impinge on the hip socket rim on attempts at external rotation. Normal femoral anteversion is approximately 40° in the newborn and usually decreases quite rapidly during the first two years of life. Fifteen degrees of anteversion is normal in older children and adults. In severe cases of femoral anteversion, surgical derotation may be necessary since there is no effective brace or shoe treatment for this problem.

External Rotation Contracture. Children in the first few months of life may exhibit a markedly externally rotated lower extremity. Examination in the supine or prone position will demonstrate the excessive external rotation and markedly diminished internal rotation of the hip. This condition is due to an abduction–external rotation contracture of the soft tissues around the hip, secondary to intrauterine position. Generally, correction will be spontaneous after the child has been on his feet and walking for several months. The parent can be instructed in exercises to stretch the posterior hip capsule by internally rotating the lower extremities when changing diapers.

Medial Tibial Torsion. In this condition the tibia is rotated medially on its long axis, causing the foot to point inward. The majority of neonates can be expected to have this positioning of their tibiae, and it seems to be related to intrauterine posture.

Most examiners use the relationship of the medial to the lateral malleolus to determine the transmalleolar axis and its relationship to the long axis of the tibia or a specific protuberance of the tibia, such as the anterior tibial tubercle. The transmalleolar axis is usually slightly rotated externally, approximately 5° in the neonate, increasing with growth to an average of 22° in the adult. The greatest increase occurs in the first 18 months of life. Lateral bowing of the tibia is a common finding in children under 18 months of age and can accentuate the appearance of internal tibial torsion.

Femoral–Tibial Angular Deformities. Mild bowing of the lower extremities (apex laterally) is a normal finding in the neonate and young child under 18 months of age. Generally, the bowing (up to 15°) is confined to the tibia (genu varum or bowleg; see Fig. 9-6A), but occasionally it can be noted in the distal femur as well. It is often accompanied by internal tibial torsion. Involvement is usually symmetrical. This condition should correct spontaneously between 18 months to 3 years of age; the child gradually develops knock-knees, or genu

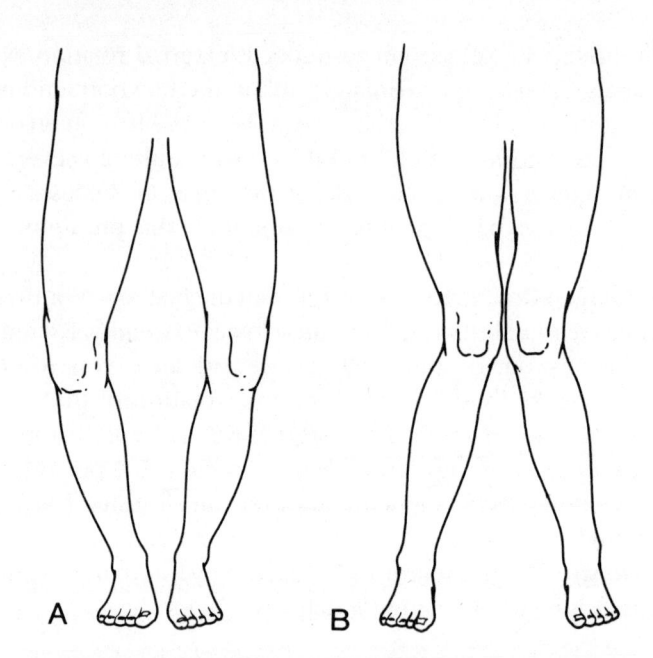

Figure 9-6. *A:* Bowlegs or genu varum. Varus is a deformity with its angle toward the midline of the body. *B:* Knock-knees or genu valgum. Valgus is a deformity with its angle away from the midline of the body.

valgum (Fig. 9-6*B*). Valgus indicates an angle away from the centerline of the body, and varus an angle toward the centerline.

Radiographically, the proximal tibia and distal femur appear to be angulated medially; the medial cortex of the tibia may be thickened, with normal appearance of the epiphyseal plate. Pathologic conditions that can lead to bowing in the infant include rickets, Blount's disease (aseptic necrosis of the medial condyle of the tibia), and metaphyseal dysplasia. These conditions can be distinguished radiographically from physiologic bowing, where the appearance of the epiphyses is abnormal.

Common Foot Problems

Metatarsus Adductus. Turning-in of the forepart of the foot, or metatarsus adductus, is found frequently in the newborn and may be related to intrauterine positioning. Many children who have metatarsus adductus also have internal tibial torsion. Diagnosis is best determined by inspecting the sole of the foot and can be easily documented by an inked footprint. The lateral border of the normal foot is straight, but in metatarsus adductus the border of the forefoot is convex, with the curve beginning at the base of the fifth metatarsal. Many (up to 90%) will spontaneously improve without specific treatment by age three. Treatment varies depending on the severity of the condition and particularly on whether the deformity is flexible (easily corrected by stretching) or fixed (not correctable by stretching). Stretching exercises, corrective shoes (built up medially to stretch the forefoot into abduction as the child steps), casts, and surgical correction have all been used. If the deformity is still present by 8 months of age, serial casts should be used. Casts should also be used in children with rigid metatarsus adductus, or those with flexible (easily passively correctable) metatarsus adductus who show progressive deformity on dorsiflexion at 4 to 6 months of age.

Clubfoot (Congenital Talipes Equinovarus). This is a common problem in the newborn and is familiar to most physicians. The foot is plantarflexed (in equinus) and turned inward (inverted or supinated), and the forefoot is bent toward the midline (adducted). The calcaneus is inverted and rotated beneath the plantarflexed talus. The navicular is medial to the head of the talus, and often the talus is prominent in the dorsolateral aspect of the foot, stretching the skin over the area. In unilateral cases, the calf is noticeably smaller and the foot shorter on the affected side.

The incidence is about 1 per 1000 live births, with a sex ratio of about 2 males to 1 female. There seems to be a multifactorial inheritance pattern. The cause of the condition is unknown. The problem may be in the soft tissues, with dislocation of the foot about the talus, or in a congenital distortion of the neck of the talus. There appear to be several pathologic variations that can have a similar clinical appearance.

The goal of treatment should be the creation of a flexible, plantigrade foot that fits a conventional shoe. For the newborn, early aggressive treatment is indicated because much can be lost by the slightest delay. Infants are more elastic during the first few days after delivery, and soft-tissue stretching and correction of deformities should begin soon after birth. Conservative management is preferred and can be expected to achieve a satisfactory result in approximately two thirds of the children. Early treatment lessens the likelihood that surgery will be required, but surgery is indicated when stretching and serial casts no longer improve the foot.

Congenital Dislocation of the Hip

Congenital dislocation of the hip (CDH) has an incidence of approximately 10 cases per 1000 live births. Early diagnosis and treatment have met with spectacular success, with approximately 96% of affected children developing radiologically and functionally normal hips. The longer the dislocation remains undiscovered and untreated, the greater the problems in returning the femoral head to its normal position within the acetabulum, and the poorer the chances of obtaining a satisfactory result. In the newborn, the diagnosis of dislocation is made by clinical examination. Routine screening for CDH should be an integral part of newborn and follow-up examinations during infancy.

Etiology

There is no single cause of CDH. Rather, the etiology is multifactorial, with both mechanical and physiologic factors on the part of the mother and infant and, occasionally, postnatal and environmental factors combining to produce hip instability and subsequent dislocation. The typical congenital dislocation occurs just prior to or following delivery in an otherwise normal infant. The mechanical factors that predispose the typical dislocation occur primarily in the last trimester of pregnancy. All have the effect of restricting the space available for the fetus in the uterus. It is believed that the pelvis of the fetus becomes trapped in the maternal pelvis. The fetus is unable to kick and change positions; thus the normal flexion of the hip and knee or limb folding is hindered. Sixty percent of children with CDH are firstborns. The tight, unstretched maternal abdominal and uterine musculature may restrict fetal movement.

Breech presentation also plays a significant role in the etiology of CDH. It is believed that breech presentation is a factor because the legs can be jackknifed (hyperflexed) in this position and thus forced out of their sockets. Thirty to fifty percent of children with CDH are delivered in this presentation. If, in addition, the knees are extended (frank breech), the increased tension in the hamstrings can further contribute to hip instability.

The left hip is more frequently involved in CDH than the right. It is believed that a fetus in the breech position tends to lie with the left thigh against the maternal sacrum. The fetal pelvis is held securely in this position, forcing the hip into a posture of flexion and adduction. In this position the femoral head is covered more by the joint capsule than by the bony acetabulum. The right hip is dislocated in 20% of patients and both hips in 25%. The incidence of CDH is increased in children who have other conditions caused by intrauterine positioning. Congenital muscular torticollis (infantile wryneck), for example, is believed to result from intrauterine compression, and up to 20% of children with this condition have associated hip instability. Also, children with deformities of the feet believed to be caused by molding, such as metatarsus adductus or calcaneal valgus, have an increased risk of CDH.

The physiologic factors in the development of CDH are the maternal estrogens and those hormones that affect pelvic relaxation just prior to delivery. Their pharmacologic effect is not limited to the maternal pelvis; it may lead to temporary laxity of the pelvic joints and hip capsule in the newborn.

Postnatal environmental factors may also contribute to the development of hip instability and dislocation. In the first months after delivery, the normal physiologic position of the hip is that of flexion and abduction. In societies where infants are customarily wrapped to a cradle board or swaddled to maintain the lower extremities in extension, the instance of congenital hip dislocation is ten times greater than normal.

Pathomechanics

The mechanism of a typical congenital dislocation is probably quite simple. Near the time of birth, the joint capsule is distended and elastic. Following delivery, the femoral head is loose within the joint and free to "fall out" of the acetabulum. If the dislocation is recognized during the newborn period, the femoral head can easily be reduced to its normal position. At this early stage, the shape of the joint and soft-tissue structures is very close to normal. Thus, for a stable hip to develop, it is only necessary to maintain a normal relationship between the femoral head and the acetabulum in the newborn for a few weeks while the joint capsule returns to its normal configuration. A deep cavelike acetabulum is an important factor in maintaining stability of

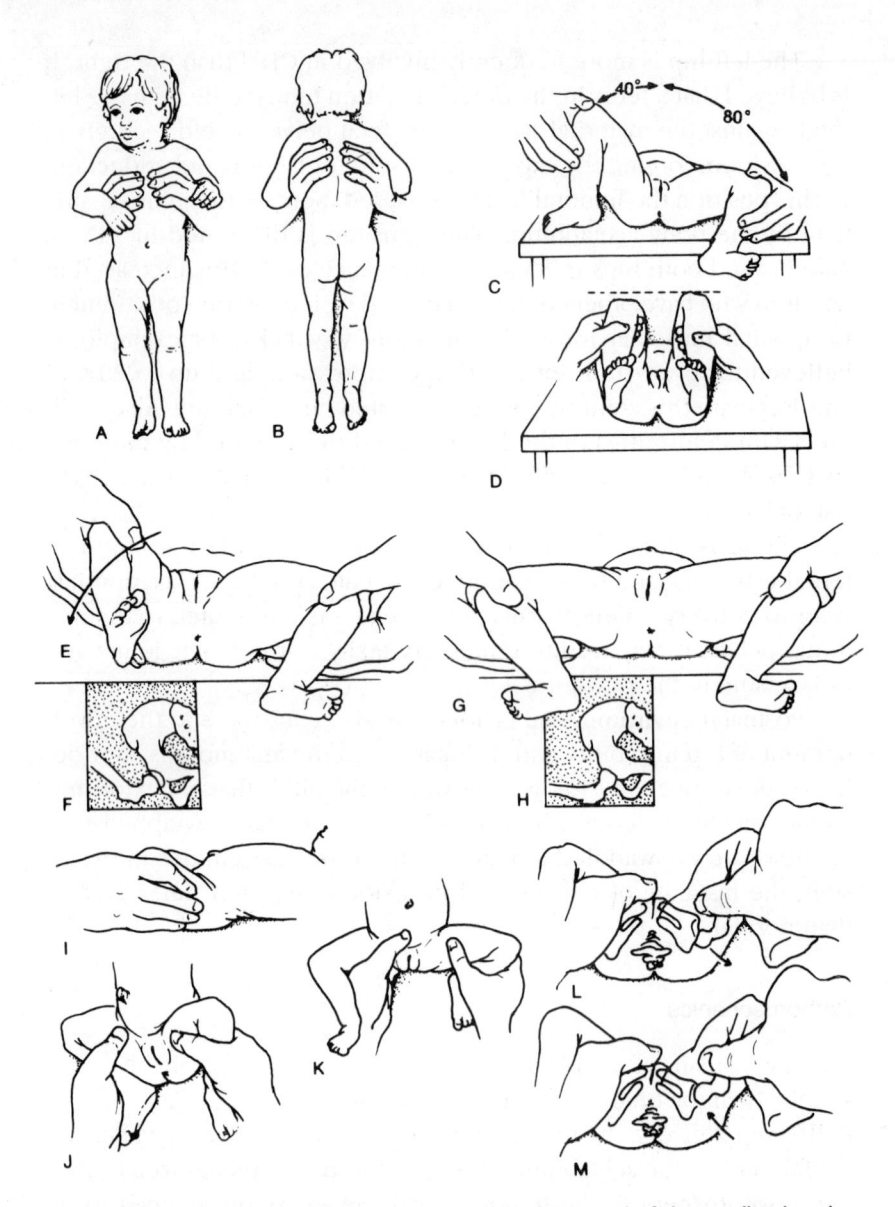

Figure 9-7. *A* and *B:* asymmetry of the thigh folds and of the popliteal and gluteal creases with apparent shortening of the extremity on the right. *C:* limited abduction of the right hip. *D:* Galleazzi's sign—apparent shortening of the femur as shown by the difference of the knee levels with the hips and knees flexed at right angles and the child lying on a firm table. *E* to *H:* Ortolani's sign—the presence of a palpable click in and out as the hip is reduced by abduction and dislocated by adduction. In insets *F* and *H* note how the femoral

the hip. The acetabulum can only develop adequate depth during growth if the femoral head is inside to "mold" it. Thus, after early reduction, the hip has the potential for remodeling into a normally shaped socket. If the dislocation is allowed to persist, however, the soft tissue and bone adjacent to the joint gradually undergo adaptive changes. The dislocation then becomes more difficult to reduce, it has to be "held" reduced longer to remodel, and the chance for obtaining a successful long-term result diminishes significantly.

Diagnosis

The most reliable method for diagnosing CDH in the newborn period is that described by Ortolani. The Ortolani examination is a test of hip reduction: when the infant with a dislocated hip is examined, the femoral head can be returned to the acetabulum with the Ortolani maneuver, demonstrating the presence of dislocation. Barlow's test is the reverse of the Ortolani maneuver. When the infant is examined, the femoral head is located within the acetabulum; however, when the hip is flexed and the thigh brought into an adducted position, the femoral head falls "or can be gently pushed" posteriorly out of the acetabulum, demonstrating an unstable hip joint (Fig. 9-7). It is common to refer to both parts of the examination collectively as the "Ortolani test." The Ortolani test should not be a forceful examination, and the infant must be relaxed and content. Cooperation by the patient and patience on the part of the examiner significantly affect the accuracy

---

head slides in across the posterior rim of the acetabulum and enters the socket as the hip is abducted. *I* to *M:* Barlow's test for the "unstable hip." The infant lies on his back with the hips flexed to 90° and the knees flexed fully. *I* and *J* show the position of the long finger of each hand over the greater trochanter and of the thumb opposite the lesser trochanter in the inner side of the upper thigh. *K* shows an alternate method used in doubtful cases. The pelvis is steadied between the thumb over the pubis and fingers under the sacrum while the hip is tested with the other hand. *L:* the hips are brought into midabduction. Thumb pressure applied posteriorly over the lesser trochanter can dislocate the femoral head across the posterior lip of the acetabulum. *M:* on release of the thumb pressure, the femoral head slips back into the acetabular socket, indicating that the hip is "unstable—not dislocated, but dislocatable." (Tachdjian MO: Pediatric Orthopedics, vol 1, pp 136–137. Philadelphia, WB Saunders, 1972)

of the examination. A child who is kicking and crying may preclude a satisfactory examination by tightening the adductors and hamstrings.

As the child grows, the clinical findings of an untreated dislocated hip become more obvious. The surrounding soft tissue and bone gradually adapt to the abnormal position of the femoral head. With time, it becomes more difficult to reduce the femoral head into the acetabulum, and the Ortolani test becomes negative. In other words, the femoral head becomes trapped outside the acetabulum. All muscle groups about the hip become shortened and contracted. Adductor tightness reflected by limited thigh abduction is most apparent. As the thigh is shortened and the skin and subcutaneous tissue bunch up, extra skin folds can be observed; with the patient supine and the knees flexed, the knees will not be at the same levels (Allis' or Galeazzi's sign; see Fig. 9-7). The femur can be freely moved up and down (described as "pistoning" and "telescoping").

X-ray Findings

Routine x-ray examination of the newborn is seldom reliable in detecting a typical congenital dislocation. Even if the hip is clinically held in a dislocated position, roentgenograms may not reveal the dislocation. The usual bony landmarks are not visible because much of the infant's pelvis is cartilaginous and consequently radiolucent. Moreover, the dislocation may be so recent that many of the pathologic changes characteristically associated with CDH will not have had sufficient time to develop and therefore will not be apparent on the film. Finally, if the femur lies in front of or behind the hip socket so as to overlap, a dislocated hip cannot be detected. Thus, a negative finding on simple anterior–posterior view cannot rule out the presence of a dislocation. Although diagnosis can be made with multiple views, particularly after the infant is dislocated with the Barlow maneuver, this is seldom practical and involves further radiation exposure.

The earliest stage at which one can reliably recognize the changes associated with a typical dislocated hip on a single roentgenogram is at approximately 6 weeks of age, because by then the secondary ossification center of the femoral head has ossified enough to be visible on x-ray (Fig. 9-8). As the child grows, the adaptive changes of the hip joint and femur become evident on routine roentgenogram. The characteristic findings from an anterior–posterior roentgenographic view of the pelvis and hips include proximal and lateral migration of

Congenital and Developmental Conditions 147

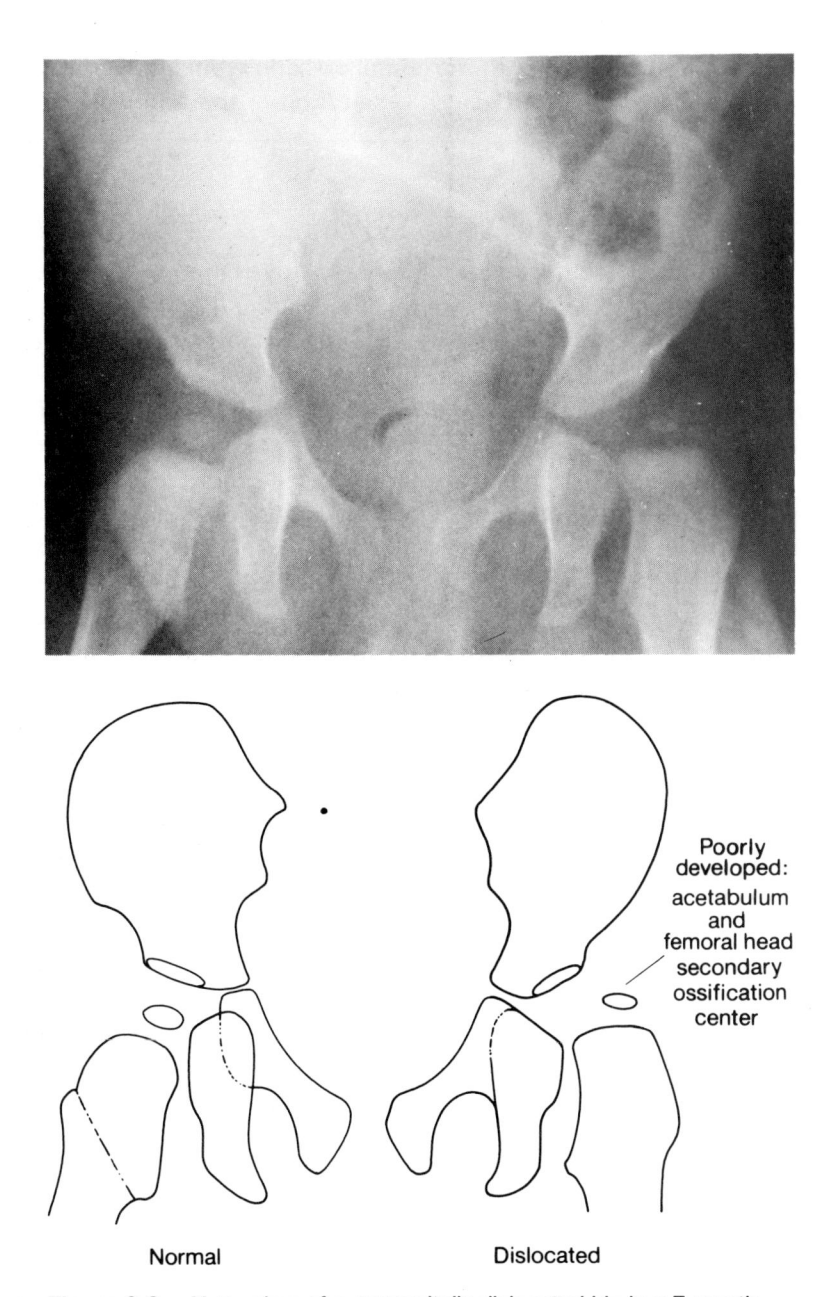

Figure 9-8. X-ray view of a congenitally dislocated hip in a 7-month-old child. The epiphysis of the femoral head is not ossified at the time of birth and thus is not well visualized by x-ray until later. The anatomic distortion effectively shortens the lever arm of the muscle that inserts on the greater trochanter and abducts the hip.

the femoral neck adjacent to the ilium, a shallow, incompletely developed acetabulum, and delayed ossification of the femoral ossific nucleus.

Treatment

In the newborn with marked instability (positive Ortolani), it is best to resort directly to a secure restraint, anticipating that the reduction will have to be maintained consistently for the joint structures to return to normal. Many restraints that maintain the hip reduced in the infant have been described, and nearly all can achieve a successful end result, provided they are properly applied and hold the femoral head reduced in a comfortable and physiologically safe position of flexion–abduction. Conversely, any restraint, if improperly applied or adjusted, can cause problems, such as redislocation or avascular necrosis of the femoral head.

The duration of treatment is directly related to the age at which treatment is begun. The earlier the dislocation is discovered, the less adaptive (pathologic) change there is to reverse, and the shorter the period needed to achieve acetabular remodeling, clinical stability, and a radiologically normal hip joint. An estimate of the period of treatment required to obtain clinically and radiologically normal hip is approximately two times the age of the child when the restraint (brace or cast) is first applied. Many orthopaedists feel that in children above 6 months of age, dislocated hips should be reduced under anesthesia, and that depending on the contracture of the surrounding tissues, cutting of the adductors or preliminary traction is indicated. In children over 18 months of age the remodeling potential is limited enough that surgical intervention with pelvis osteotomy to shift the position of the socket is frequently indicated. Above the age of 4 or 5, even with reduction, the remodeling will frequently be inadequate and result in hips that are not congruently concentric. This may lead to hip arthrosis in later years.

Chapter 10

The Limping Child

Eric T. Jones

Limping is never normal. It can be caused by something as simple as a stone in the shoe, but it can also be the first manifestation of an osteogenic sarcoma or chronic renal disease. A discussion of limp must cover the important musculoskeletal conditions affecting children of walking age, but it should also reveal the broad spectrum of problems that must be considered when evaluating a child with a skeletal complaint.

Normal walking or running is rhythmic and seemingly effortless. The child's center of gravity shifts back and forth over the lower extremities so quickly and smoothly that the pelvis and trunk seem to remain stationary. To critically assess a limp or an abnormal gait, it is first necessary to understand this normal pattern, and the best method of studying normal gait is to observe the child performing a variety of activities. In the office setting, it is usual practice to watch the child walk or run for a short distance. A discussion of gait is, by necessity, limited to guidelines for better observation.

A child's motor skills and ability to ambulate constantly improve because the child's central nervous system is maturing and the child is gaining more experience. Most children are able to stand unassisted and begin walking by the time they are one year old. More-complex activities, such as being able to walk up and down steps and being able to balance on one foot, may not take place until the child is two or three years old. Usually a child is at least three years of age before he walks in the adult heel–toe pattern.

Components of Gait

Gait can be divided into two phases: stance and swing. During the stance phase, the foot is in contact with the floor and this limb bears the body weight. Stance phase begins with heel strike and ends with toe off. A short stance phase is characteristic of an antalgic gait, as the child quickly vaults over the extremity that hurts. During the swing phase, the foot does not touch the floor. This phase begins with toe off and ends with heel strike. A child with stiff hip has a short swing phase due to the limited flexion of the hip joint.

Hip and Pelvis

The pelvis normally rotates forward and tilts a small amount during swing phase. The trunk normally maintains a neutral position and excessive motion usually signals a problem. If hip joint motion is limited, it is necessary for the pelvis and trunk to be thrust further forward to accomplish the same degree of progression. Elevation of the pelvis may occur in swing phase to gain more clearance for a stiff hip or knee. If a limb is short, the pelvis and trunk will fall more to that side during stance phase.

Gluteus Medius Limp (Trendelenburg Gait). When a normal child stands on one leg, the gluteus medius on the same side maintains the opposite side of the pelvis level by pulling from the top of the pelvis to the greater trochanter. If the gluteus medius is weak, the opposite side of the pelvis dips down during stance phase (a positive Trendelenburg sign; Fig. 10-1). With each step, the child's trunk may shift toward the side of a painful or weak extremity in order to decrease the force transmitted through the extremity. This may happen so rapidly that one observes only a lurch of the trunk or a dip of the pelvis. Bilateral involvement results in a waddling gait.

Congenital dislocation of the hip destroys the normal center of rotation of the hip, effectively shortening the lever arm of the gluteus medius muscle and substantially weakening it (see Fig. 9-8). This is a common cause of a Trendelenburg limp.

Gluteus Maximus Limp. In the absence of the gluteus maximus, a powerful hip extensor, the patient leans backward to balance the trunk over the pelvis (Fig. 10-2). This is characteristic of conditions that

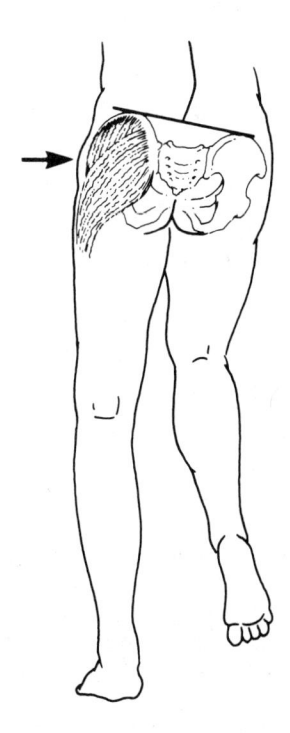

Figure 10-1. Drawing depicts a positive Trendelenburg sign. During the single-leg stance phase weak hip abductors cannot hold the pelvis level.

cause proximal muscle weakness, such as muscular dystrophy, or spine problems that cause hip muscle weakness.

Knee

The knee normally flexes about 70° during swing phase. If it is unable to flex, the child will have to elevate the pelvis and swing the leg outward or circumduct the extremity for the foot to clear the floor. Problems related to the foot and ankle can also cause alteration of knee motion. Lack of ankle dorsiflexion or a drop foot (as may be seen after polio or Charcot-Marie-Tooth disease, or as associated with clubfoot or cerebral palsy) necessitates a greater degree of knee flexion during swing phase in order for the toes to clear. This is commonly called a "steppage gait."

An equinus deformity (fixed plantar flexion of the ankle) functionally lengthens the extremity (Fig. 10-3). Compensation is commonly accomplished by incomplete knee and hip extension in the stance phase of gait. Hyperextension of knee ("back-kneeing" or *recurvatum*) during stance phase is generally the result of relative in-

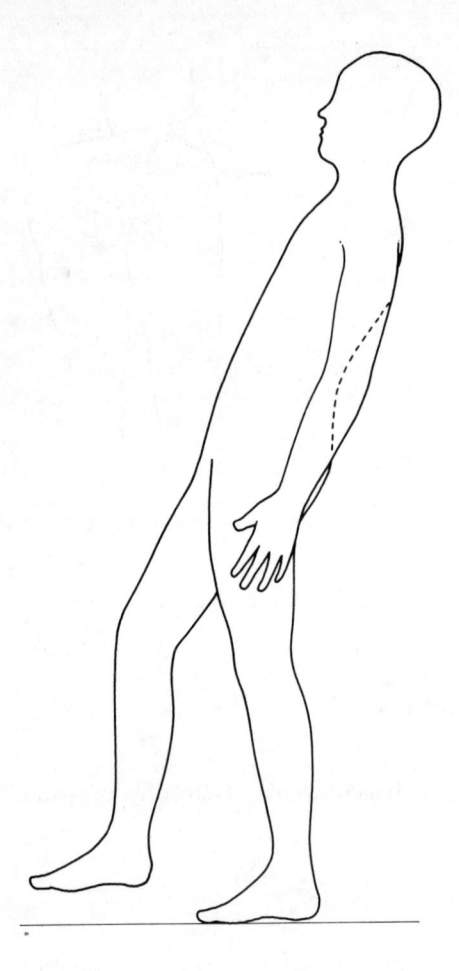

Figure 10-2. In single-leg stance, weakness of the gluteus maximus causes the patient to lean backward in order to balance the upper torso over the pelvis.

stability of the knee frequently caused by muscle weakness about the knee. The knee is more stable in the extended position than when flexed; back-kneeing represents a compensatory measure to gain stability.

Quadriceps Femoris Limp. Weakness of the quadriceps femoris is associated with a near-normal gait on level ground, as long as the child walks slowly. The critical observer should detect a little more backknee as the child locks the knee in extension during stance phase and elevates the pelvis on the opposite side to vault over this weakened extremity. Weakness limits the climbing of stairs. Frequently the child will use the hand on the thigh to help push up the stairs (Fig. 10-4).

The Limping Child   153

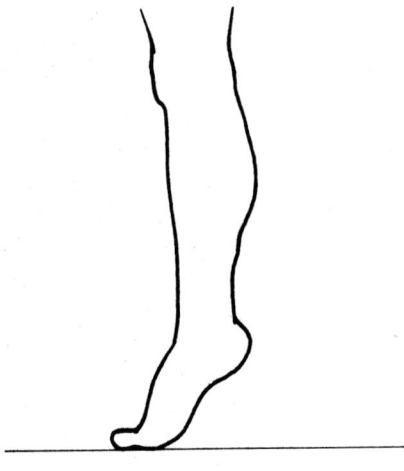

Figure 10-3. In equinus deformity, the foot is in fixed plantar flexion, much like the hoof of a horse.

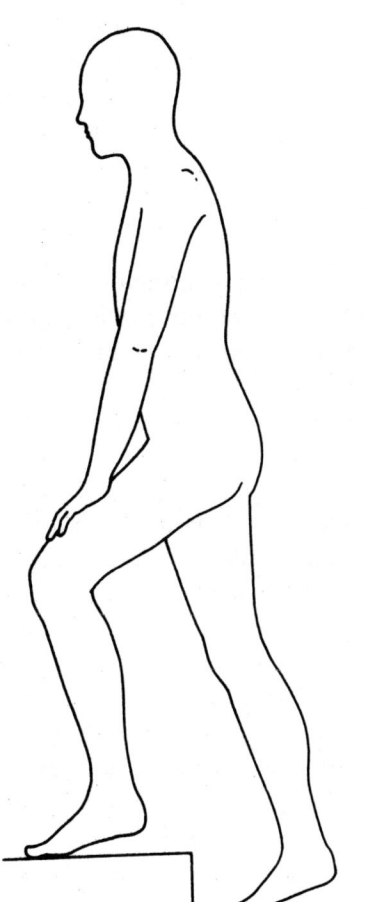

Figure 10-4. An individual with weakness of the quadriceps femoris can mask the deformity by stabilizing the knee in gait with careful adjustment of the center of gravity over the stance leg. However, the weakness becomes apparent when the individual tries to go up stairs and has to push the knee into extension with his hand.

Foot and Ankle

Approximately 10° of dorsiflexion and 20° of plantar flexion of the ankles are necessary for normal gait. If plantar flexion is restricted (*e.g.,* from a tight heel cord), there is no push-off onto the toes at the end of the stance phase. The forefoot and heel come off the floor at the same time. Lack of dorsiflexion causes the foot to hang down during swing phase and forces the knee to lift higher (the steppage gait mentioned above) or the toes to drag on the floor ("drop foot"). In this situation, the accessory muscles of dorsiflexion play a greater role in trying to dorsiflex the foot, and the now-unopposed muscles of the foot may pull the toes into a clawed position. This is commonly seen in the older child with Charcot-Marie-Tooth disease or in spine problems such as myelodysplasia where there is distal weakness. With dorsiflexion weakness, smooth deceleration of the foot cannot be controlled and the forefoot slaps against the floor. Toe walking may result from spasticity, as in cerebral palsy, contracture of the gastroc-soleus group, or simply from attempts to compensate for a short extremity.

History

The exact circumstances surrounding the onset and duration of a limp must be carefully explored. An episode of trauma should be investigated; however, a seemingly innocuous incident associated with very little trauma may cause a fracture through bone weakened by a preexisting tumor. There are a number of points to be considered; for example, is the limp always there, or is it only transient? Does it occur only in the morning or at the end of the day? Does it occur when the child is tired, with activity, or is it there throughout the day? The physician should bear in mind that a young child who limps may refuse to walk or stand at all and ask to be carried. What is the posture of the lower extremity when the child is limping? What is the effect of stair climbing or running? Limping after vigorous activity may be the first clue to an impending stress fracture.

If pain is associated with the limp, the exact location and pattern of the pain should be ascertained. Pain from the low back is referred to the buttocks and lateral thigh, whereas pain from the hip joint is more often localized to the groin or "referred" to the inner aspect of the thigh or knee. The pattern of referred pain in children seems to be stronger than in adults. An excellent example is pain referred to the knee from the hip. With problems about the medial aspect of the hip joint, such as slipped capital femoral epiphysis or tumors in the trochanteric region of the hip joint, the child will usually complain of "knee pain." It is also helpful to know the character of the pain. Constant pain may be the result of an expanding tumor; pain at night suggests an inflammatory lesion or tumor. Pain associated with joint motion is highly suggestive of interarticular disturbances. Conditions leading to demineralization of bone, such as rickets, frequently cause generalized pain, particularly in the weight-bearing bones of the lower extremity. Limping may be the first sign of systemic illness, such as acute leukemia, storage diseases (such as Gaucher's disease), or chronic renal disease.

The age of the patient may lead the physician to suspect certain conditions. In the child who is just beginning to walk, up to 18 months or 2 years of age, hip dysplasia is the most common cause of limp. Painless limp in a young child can be caused by congenital dislocation of the hip. A waddling gait is associated with bilaterally dislocated hips, while the more remarkable Trendelenburg limp suggests a unilateral congenitally dislocated hip. A child with cerebral palsy will characteristically have a tight heel cord and dynamic inturning of his lower extremity, and may present with limp. Likewise, any condition that leads to weakness of the extremity, such as polio or muscular dystrophy, and any congenital limb deficiency that a child might have will present with a painless limp early in the walking years.

A painful limp in the younger child (1 to 3 years of age) may be due to infection. Osteomyelitis or septic arthritis of the hip or knee should be considered in this age group.

A child in the 3- to 5-year-old age range can have any of the conditions mentioned above for younger children, but the two most common conditions that cause limp in this age group are *Perthes' disease* and transient synovitis of the hip. Perthes' disease is osteonecrosis of the femoral head and was really described simultaneously by three physicians: Legg of Boston, Calvé of France, and Perthes of Germany. Osteonecrosis of the femoral head is a better and more descriptive term. This condition is more common in boys; physical examination usually reveals tightness and spasm of the adductor muscles. It can be diagnosed by the clinical findings and x-ray views that show increased density of the dead femoral head. In a growing child the blood supply to the femoral head enters the epiphysis through the epiphyseal vessels. (There are no blood vessels through the epiphyseal center while it is open.) These vessels are extra-articular; they are also embedded in delicate and fragile connective tissue in the femoral neck. There is also a blood vessel that enters the femoral head from the acetabular side through the ligamentum teres. Although there is no conclusive agreement as to what causes Legg–Perthes' disease, it may result, in the growing child, from transient swelling with effusion of the hip joint capsule which shuts off the extra-articular blood vessels to the femoral head. There is also some discussion about the role of the artery of the ligamentum teres in supplying blood to the femoral head throughout growth. It has been suggested that the period from 4 to 6 or 7 years of age is a critical time when the blood supply to the femoral head is tenuous because the ligamentum teres vessel becomes less important and the remaining blood supply is thus subject to occlusion. Whatever the cause, the result is that the bone of the femoral head dies and is revascularized. During this process of revascularization and the remodeling of the femoral head with new bone, the bone is somewhat plastic and easily deformable. Thus, normal load on this bone during the healing period can lead to flattening and misshaping of the femoral head.

Transient synovitis, probably the most common cause of painful hip in children under 10 years of age, is the term given to synovitis with effusion of the hip, which appears to be related to trauma to that joint. The condition can present itself suddenly and can be difficult to distinguish from infection. Why children and not adults tend to develop this condition is not well understood. There is always limitation of motion of the hip, and the lower extremity may be held in a flexed, abducted posture similar to the posture that occurs with septic arthritis of the hip. Many children will present with spasm about the hip and pain on motion that last just a few days and then resolve spontaneously without any subsequent x-ray evidence of osteonecrosis. These children frequently have a preexisting upper-respiratory-tract infection. They usually do not look septic. Nor do they have high fevers or high white blood cell counts, but they may have a minimally elevated sedimentation rate. The only way to be sure that there is no infection present is to aspirate joint fluid. There is no statistical relationship between transient synovitis of the hip and osteonecrosis of the femoral head, although many believe that a relationship does exist.

Other causes of limp in this age group are disc-space infection, or spinal cord, pelvic, or lower extremity tumors. The most common benign tumors in childhood are unicameral bone cysts, osteoid osteomas, and eosinophilic granulomas. The most common malignant tumors are Ewing's sarcoma and osteogenic sarcoma.

In the older child (10 to 12 years of age), *slipped capital femoral epiphysis* may also be a cause for limp. This characteristically occurs in the obese, hypogonadal child. External rotation and shortening of the extremity are usually present. The condition may present itself suddenly or chronically, with medial thigh or knee pain and limp as the presenting complaints. The capital of the femoral epiphysis is the center responsible for the growth of the femoral head and is the portion of the proximal femur that contributes to the longitudinal growth of that bone. The epiphysis sits at a bit of an angle to the horizontal and is subject to shear stress and subsequent fracture. When it fractures, it displaces medially and somewhat posteriorly. The patient complains of pain (frequently at the knee!), and the fracture is associated with blood in the joint and a subsequent synovitis.

Spondylolisthesis, a congenital or acquired absence of or fracture through the pars interarticularis allowing forward slippage of the proximal vertebra over the distal one, can also lead to an abnormal gait in this age group. Charcot-Marie-Tooth disease, with distal weakness, can also cause children to limp; these children classically have a "drop foot."

Problems in the foot that result in a limp are characteristically present in the 10- to 12-year-old. Since the conditions are present from birth, it is a little unclear why these patients wait so long to manifest a limp. It would appear, though, that at about the age of 12 or 13 the foot, because its growth has stopped for the most part, becomes more rigid. Thus the children are less able to compensate for their congenital abnormalities. The more common conditions include area tarsal coalitions (congenital fusion of the hind foot bones), accessory navicular, and osteonecrosis of bones in the foot. These can usually be diagnosed radiographically.

Stress-related conditions in the region of the knee can cause growing children to limp. The most common of these are Osgood–Schlatter disease (avulsion of the tibial tubercle), jumper's knee (patellar tendonitis), and patellofemoral tracking problems.

Important in children of all ages are seasonal complaints such as those that appear in the springtime when children are returning to activities outdoors and may not have been active for some time. Stress fractures occur from the failure of muscles to protect the bone from repetitive stress. Although there is no clear supporting evidence, there has been some suggestion that heel pain is caused by small microinjuries to the epiphyseal plate of the calcaneus. Thus heal pain may be another common complaint associated with limp in the growing child.

Besides osteomyelitis and septic arthritis, other inflammatory conditions that must be considered are conditions, such as juvenile arthritis, that can occur in any age range but are probably more common in the 5- to 12-year-old range.

Physical Examination

The physician should ask the child to walk in front of him several times until he is able to determine the abnormality in the child's gait. The child should be asked, while walking, to say if and when he feels pain, and the parent should be asked to point out the various abnormalities because the parent is familiar with the child's normal gait. Limitation of the range of motion of a single joint forces joints on either side to move with greater excursion to make up for the lack of motion. This can result in an irregular and jerky gait that may be confusing until one has watched a number of children walk. Moreover, the rotational position of the extremity may change; for example, the external rotation may adapt to accommodate a stiff ankle with limited dorsiflexion or a slipped capital femoral epiphysis. Often it is helpful to observe the function of isolated muscle groups by having the child walk up on his toes or heels or try to climb stairs.

Slapping of the foot in a patient with a foot drop or the scraping type of walk sometimes associated with a spastic gait can yield important information. Also, the physician should note the variations in time between the two sides in stance phase, since quick steps in gait can indicate pain. Sometimes inspecting the shoes for abnormal wear can indicate where the problem lies.

Static examination of the child on the examining table should clarify impressions gained while watching the child walk. The joints should be examined individually and compared with the opposing joints to discover any limitation of motion or guarding. Limb length can best be evaluated by having the child stand and leveling his pelvis by placing blocks beneath the foot of the shorter extremity. Observation and girth measurement for atrophy can be helpful to identify the location of a problem.

In children presenting with pain in the knee, if the knee examination is normal, it is important to remember to check for range of motion of the hip, since hip problems commonly present with knee pain.

A complete neurologic examination, including testing for strength and deep-tendon reflexes, is important because weakness secondary to spine problems can present itself as a limp.

Laboratory Studies

The history and physical examination are probably the most important means of identifying the cause of the limp. This information, in combination with the child's age, should allow the physician to make a good guess as to what the child's problem is. Radiographic examination may be the way to confirm that diagnosis. In young children, the best radiographic examination is an anterior–posterior view of both lower extremities with the child standing. In older children with a painful limp, the physician can usually determine which x-ray studies are indicated. Osteomyelitis and septic arthritis may not show abnormalities on film, and these conditions are more often diagnosed early by history and physical examination. A bone scan may demonstrate the early inflammation of osteomyelitis or disc-space infection. Laboratory studies, including blood count with differential, sedimentation rate, and blood cultures, are important; however, the most important laboratory study is probably direct aspiration of a joint with fluid in it. This can often establish the diagnosis and the cause of the limp.

Chapter 11

Scoliosis

Eric T. Jones

Scoliosis, a deviation in the normally straight vertical line of the spine, occurs with an incidence of about 20 cases per 1000 in which the deviation is greater than 10°. Idiopathic scoliosis accounts for about 85% of all cases, and congenital deformity accounts for most of the remainder. Not all cases of idiopathic scoliosis are progressive; therefore, not all patients require treatment. There is no known method, however, for predicting when scoliosis will be progressive. The incidence in males and females is identical, although progressive curvature and curves requiring treatment are about 7 times more common in females than in males. If the deviation progresses, it is likely to do so during the rapid growth of adolescence.

Limb-length discrepancy can be a major cause of small lumbar curves, and this should be sought. Approximately 80% of patients with idiopathic scoliosis present with a positive family history; siblings of patients should be screened. Idiopathic scoliosis appears to be inherited in a multifactorial fashion, but in some families it behaves as a dominant trait. Although dramatic scoliosis usually occurs in adolescence, as noted, progression may sometimes continue throughout adulthood, with one to two additional degrees of deviation added each year.

Scoliosis is characterized by lateral deviation of the spinal column and rotational deviation of the involved vertebrae (Fig. 11-1). The rotation is due to the fact that lateral and axial rotations of the vertebral bodies are coupled actions. The anatomy dictates that rotation in the frontal plane cannot happen without rotation in the cross-sectional

162 Pediatric Orthopaedic Problems

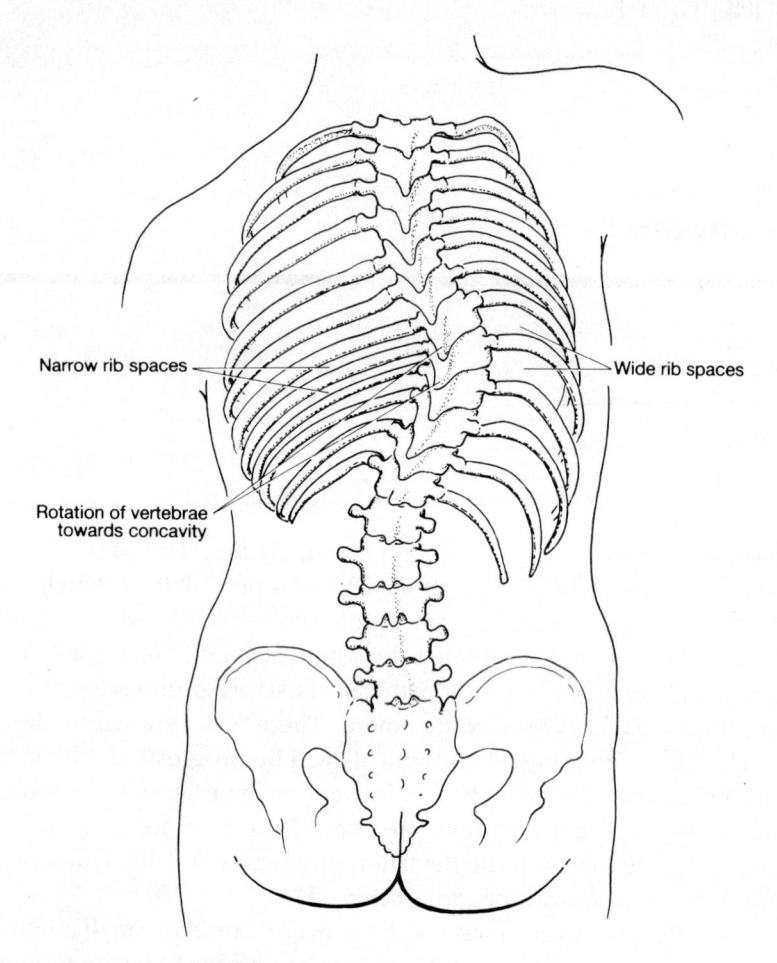

Figure 11-1. Scoliosis with a thoracic curve. Note the axial rotation of the vertebral bodies and the associated rib deformities.

plane. The rib hump occurs because the ribs articulate with the thoracic vertebral bodies. When these costovertebral joints are rotated, the ribs protrude posteriorly on one side. The most commonly involved vertebrae are the thoracic, which usually form a curve to the right of normal position. In this instance the thoracic vertebrae are rotated clockwise as viewed from the top of the spinal column, or to the left as viewed posteriorly. When the curve is to the right, the ribs rotate posteriorly on the right side, and the ribs on the left are crowded together in the concavity. The affected vertebrae become wedge-shaped, and disc spaces on the left are narrowed.

Severe deformities of the spine significantly decrease pulmonary function. Pulmonary complications occur in those patients with curves greater than 60° or with thoracic lordosis. In patients above age 50 with curves greater than 90°, the risk of death is 3 times greater, and a working disability is 20 times more likely. A 50% reduction in vital capacity may occur in curves over 60°.

Examination for scoliosis includes physical and radiographic components. Physical examination may show asymmetry in the waist line, in the airspace between the arms and waistline, in the shoulder and neck lines, and in scapular prominence. Upon forward bending, viewed posteriorly, the rib cage and lumbar area may be prominent on one side (Fig. 11-2A, B). Other abnormalities that may be evident are kyphosis or abnormal lordosis; these findings may be apparent in the absence or presence of scoliosis. The only x-ray view appropriate for the primary physician to order is a single standing posterior–anterior spine film, unless kyphosis or lordosis is clearly present. A lateral view radiograph involves a high amount of radiation and is best obtained in a referral situation. Determination of whether scoliosis is idiopathic or congenital can be made radiographically, by seeking the deformed or partially formed vertebra of congenital scoliosis. Scoliosis is not painful; other problems such as infection, tumors, spondylolysis, or spondylolisthesis should be considered and investigated if pain is present.

Treatment depends on the severity of the disorder and, most important, on the skeletal maturity of the patient. By age one, 50% of the total growth of the spine has occurred. This is an important consideration in the management of congenital spinal deformity, particularly in the young child. A short-segment spinal fusion (bony bridging of intervertebral joints) is not as stunting to the ultimate height of the child as is bony fusion of the growth plates of the lower extremities. In addition, in children with congenital abnormal spinal curvature (scoliosis or kyphosis), the spine growth may not be straight and, thus, does not contribute to longitudinal growth, but rather to growth in a pathologic direction. The spinal cord stays approximately the same length during the period of spinal column growth, so the neural elements effectively migrate in a cephalad direction. In the older child the spinal cord ends at about L1. Most idiopathic scoliosis is nonpro-

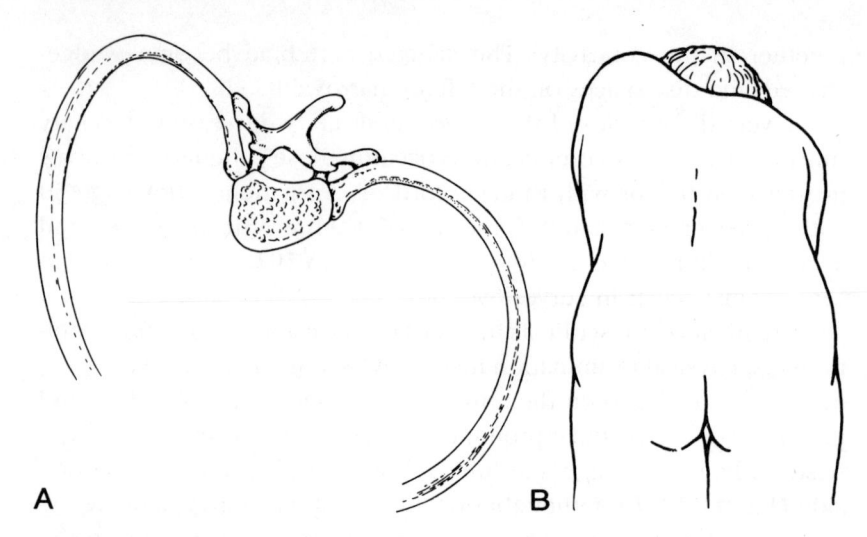

Figure 11-2. *A:* A cross section of a thorax with scoliosis. Note the distortion of the vertebrae and ribs. *B:* View of the back of a patient with scoliosis who is bending forward showing the prominent rib hump.

gressive and does not require treatment. The later the scoliosis starts in a child's life, the less likely it is to progress. If curvature starts early, it is likely that scoliosis will be progressive and will result in a more severe curvature. The greater the angle of the curve when it is initially detected, the greater the likelihood that it will progress. Curves less than 30° have about a 20% risk of increase, and curves greater than 50° have about a 90% risk of increasing if the patient is skeletally immature.

If progressive scoliosis is detected early, progression may be halted with use of a brace. Generally patients with curves in the 20° to 40° range are braced if their condition is progressive; curves of a lesser degree will be braced if the patient is skeletally immature or if there is reason to believe that the scoliosis is progressive. It is important for the patient's family and for the primary physician to understand that brace treatment, if needed, does not improve the curvature, but negates its progression. Patients with curves greater than 50° to 60° are not candidates for brace treatment and may require surgery. Severe curves can be stabilized with surgery, that is, spinal fusion, with or without the insertion of fixation rods, which can be used to help straighten the curve to some extent.

Scoliosis becomes evident in children in the age range of 10 to 12 years. This is a time when children go for long periods of time without medical examination, because they are rarely sick. Many of them feel they have outgrown pediatricians and are reluctant to see a new physician unless absolutely necessary. Scoliosis is not painful and so may not be called to the patient's or physician's attention until late in the problem.

Because it is easier to treat idiopathic scoliosis if it is recognized early, some localities have adopted school screening programs. Besides the spinal curvature, which is sometimes difficult to appreciate, symptoms sought in the clinics include unlevel shoulders, a tilted pelvis, or a "rib hump." Young people treated for scoliosis in the early stages can expect to have a spine that functions virtually normally, to be able to participate in all physical activities, and to have only a minimal cosmetic deformity. The earlier treatment begins, the easier it is to get results that are acceptable, both functionally and cosmetically.

Selected Readings

Chapter One
History and Physical and Radiographic Examinations

Hoppenfeld S: Physical Examination of the Spine and Extremities. New York, Appleton-Century-Crofts, 1976

Chapter Two
Fractures and Dislocations

Aegerter E, Kirkpatrick JA: Orthopedic Diseases, 4th ed. Philadelphia, WB Saunders, 1975
Albright JA, Brand RA: The Scientific Basis of Orthopaedics. New York, Appleton-Century-Crofts, 1979
Ham AW, Cormack DH: Histology, 8th ed. Philadelphia, JB Lippincott, 1979
Ramamurti CP: Orthopaedics in Primary Care. Baltimore, Williams & Wilkins, 1979
Rockwood CA, Green DP: Fractures in Adults, 2nd ed, vol 1. Philadelphia, JB Lippincott, 1984

Chapter Three
Injuries of the Hand

American Society for Surgery of the Hand: The Hand: Examination and Diagnosis, 2nd ed. New York, Churchill Livingstone, 1983
American Society for Surgery of the Hand: The Hand: Primary Care of Common Problems. Aurora, Colo, American Society for Surgery of the Hand, 1985
Carter PR: Common Hand Injuries and Infections: A Practical Approach to Early Treatment. Philadelphia, WB Saunders, 1983

Chapter Four
Injuries of the Neck

Apley AG, Soloman L: Apley's System of Orthopaedics and Fractures, 6th ed, chap 17. Boston, Butterworth Scientific, 1982
Newmeyer WL: Primary Care of Hand Injuries. Philadelphia, Lea & Febiger, 1979
Omer GE Jr, Spinner M: Management of Peripheral Nerve Problems. Philadelphia, WB Saunders, 1980

Chapter Five
Sports Injuries

American Academy of Orthopedic Surgeons Symposium on Sports Medicine. Saint Louis, CV Mosby, 1969
Radin EL, Simon SR, Rose RM, Paul IL: Practical Biomechanics for the Orthopedic Surgeon. Chap 3. New York, John Wiley & Sons, 1979

Chapter Six
Reaction of Bone to Tumors and Infections

Aegerter E, Kirkpatrick JA: Orthopedic Diseases, 4th ed. Philadelphia, WB Saunders, 1975
Bullough PG, Vigorita VJ: Atlas of Orthopaedic Pathology. Baltimore, University Park Press, 1984
Enneking WF: Musculoskeletal Tumor Surgery. New York, Churchill Livingstone, 1983

Chapter Seven
Arthritis and Arthrosis

Aegerter E, Kirkpatrick JA: Orthopedic Diseases, 4th ed. Philadelphia, WB Saunders, 1975
Freeman MAR: Adult Articular Cartilage. New York, Grune & Stratton, 1972
Meisel AD, Bullough PG: Atlas of Osteoarthritis. Philadelphia, Lea & Febiger, 1984
Radin EL, Simon SR, Rose RM, Paul IL: Practical Biomechanics for the Orthopedic Surgeon. Chap 4. New York, John Wiley & Sons, 1979
Rodan GP, Schumacher HR: Primer on the Rheumatic Diseases, 8th ed. Atlanta, Arthritis Foundation, 1983
Sokoloff L: The Biology of Degenerative Joint Disease. Chicago, University of Chicago Press, 1969

Chapter Eight
Pain in the Back and Leg

Aegerter E, Kirkpatrick JA: Orthopedic Diseases, 4th ed. Philadelphia, WB Saunders, 1975
Farfan HF: Mechanical Disorders of the Low Back. Philadelphia, Lea & Febiger, 1973
White AA, Gordon SL: American Academy of Orthopaedic Surgeons Symposium on Idiopathic Low Back Pain. Saint Louis, CV Mosby, 1982

Chapter Nine
Congenital and Developmental Conditions

Aegerter E, Kirkpatrick JA: Orthopedic Diseases, 4th ed. Philadelphia, WB Saunders, 1975
Lovell WW, Winter RB: Pediatric Orthopaedics, 2nd ed. Philadelphia, JB Lippincott, 1986
Tachdjian MO: Pediatric Orthopedics. Philadelphia, WB Saunders, 1972

Chapter Ten
The Limping Child

Aegerter E, Kirkpatrick JA: Orthopedic Diseases, 4th ed. Philadelphia, WB Saunders, 1975
Lovell WW, Winter RB: Pediatric Orthopaedics, 2nd ed. Philadelphia, JB Lippincott, 1986
Tachdjian MO: Pediatric Orthopedics. Philadelphia, WB Saunders, 1972

Chapter Eleven
Scoliosis

Aegerter E, Kirkpatrick JA: Orthopedic Diseases, 4th ed. Philadelphia, WB Saunders, 1975
Lovell WW, Winter RB: Pediatric Orthopaedics, 2nd ed. Philadelphia, JB Lippincott, 1986
Tachdjian MO: Pediatric Orthopedics. Philadelphia, WB Saunders, 1972

Glossary

abduction The movement of a body segment away from the midline of the body, such as lifting the arm away from the side of the chest or lifting the leg out toward the side.

acetabulum The socket of the hip joint.

Achilles tendon The heel cord. It is the tendon of the calf muscles.

acromioclavicular joint The joint at the outer end of the collar bone (clavicle). The acromion is an anterior projection of the shoulder blade, and the acromioclavicular joint is the "point" of the shoulder. Separation of this joint is referred to as a "separated shoulder." "Dislocated shoulder" refers to a dislocation of the glenohumeral joint.

adduction Movement of a body segment toward the midline of the body, such as bringing the thighs close together.

anatomically neutral position Standing with arms at the sides, palms and feet forward.

annulus fibrosus *See* disc or intervertebral disc.

anterior tibial tubercle The bony prominence just under the kneecap on which the patellar tendon is inserted.

antigen–antibody response The molecular basis of the immunologic response. An antigen can be any foreign protein such as a virus or bacteria. Antibodies are produced by the host in response to an antigen. At the cellular level, the antibody attaches itself to the antigen, rendering the antigen neutral.

arteriography Injection of radiopaque material into arteries, which makes the inside of the arteries visible by x-ray.

arthrodesis *See* fusion.

arthrogram Visualization of the internal structures of the knee obtained by radiographic examination of the knee after it has been injected with radiopaque constrast material.

arthroscopic examination Examination of a joint by inserting a thin viewing tube containing a light source and appropriate optics.

articular cartilage *See* cartilage.

bipartite patellas Hereditary two-part kneecaps.

calcaneus The heel bone.

callus The calcified tissue that forms about a fracture to provide early stabilization.

cancellous bone Relatively porous bony tissue that makes up the end of bones. It is a series of interconnected, walled spaces filled with marrow. This type of bone can be considered a "honeycomb" of small interconnected bony plates and struts.

carcinoma A form of cancer.

cartilage A fiber-reinforced gel used for flexible rigidity (*e.g.*, in the ears and nose), as a low-friction bearing surface (*e.g.*, in joints), or as an intermediate phase in the formation of bone (*e.g.*, in endochondral bone formation).

cauda equina Extension of the spinal cord into the lumbar spinal canal.

center of gravity The center of an object's mass. For analytical purposes, it can be assumed that the body's weight acts from its center of gravity. In man it is a point just in front of the sacrum.

cervical radiculitis Pain in the upper extremity caused by the pinching of a nerve root in the cervical spine (neck). Nerves that serve the upper extremity emerge from the spinal cord in the neck.

Charcot-Marie-Tooth disease A slowly progressive muscle disease that usually starts in the feet and ankles and is associated with weakness and the development of deformities secondary to this weakness.

claudication Pain that comes on after walking some distance. If the patient stops, the pain goes away only to recur when the patient walks the critical distance again.

clubfoot A combination of metatarsus adductus (forefoot inversion), equinus (toes down), and varus (inversion) of the heel.

Colles' fracture Fracture involving the distal end of the radius (and sometimes ulna) caused by a fall on an outstretched hand. The wrist and hand are displaced dorsally, giving the appearance of a dislocation to the wrist with the hand displaced backward. Described by Abraham Colles, an Irish surgeon in the early 19th century, it is the most common fracture in man.

comminuted fracture Broken into many pieces.

congenital Something one is born with.

cortical bone The bony tissue that makes up the shaft of a bone. Although it contains holes for blood vessels, cortical bone is not usually very porous.

CT scan (computed tomography) Computer reconstruction of x-ray views taken from multiple projections to provide a cross-sectional view.

cuboid Small bone of the midfoot, just in front of the calcaneus (heel bone).

degenerative joint change *See* osteoarthrosis.

delayed union and nonunion There can be no general time period for defining normal fracture healing because such healing depends upon the bone involved and the degree of associated soft-tissue damage. One usually defines a *delayed union* as fracture healing that exceeds the normal expected average fracture healing time. A nonunion is a fracture that has not healed within three times the normal average healing time.

diaphysis *See* metaphysis.

diarthrodial joint A joint that contains a fluid lubricant and readily articulates.

disc or intervertebral disc The soft-tissue cushion or "bumper" between the vertebral bodies. It is composed of a gelatinous center surrounded by a fibrous ring. When a disc ruptures, the central gelatinous material comes out through a tear in the peripheral annular ring. If this tear is posterior, the ruptured disc material can press on the nerve root.

distal *See* proximal and distal.

distal interphalangeal joint *See* finger joints.

dorsal Anatomically, the back (posterior) side of the body.

dorsiflexion The act of bringing the ankle or wrist up (from the anatomically neutral position).

edema Swelling caused by increased amounts of fluid in the tissues.

effusion Fluid within a joint (*e.g.,* water on the knee).

endochondral bone formation *See* intramembranous and endochondral bone formation.

enzyme A molecule capable of digesting another molecule.

epiphysis *See* metaphysis.

equinus A contracture of the ankle such that the foot is permanently pointed downward.

extension *See* flexion and extension.

external rotation *See* internal and external rotation.

facet joints Small joints behind the vertebral bodies that articulate the back bones.

fiber bone New bone whose fibrous component is not well ordered at the microscopic level. Bone is composed of a calcified fibrous matrix. Although the matrix is always well ordered at the submicroscopic level, it need not be at the microscopic level. "Immature bone" is fiber bone.

finger joints The joint at the end of the finger is the distal interphalangeal joint (DIP), and the joint in the middle is the proximal interphalangeal joint (PIP). The juncture of the finger with the hand is the metacarpophalangeal joint (MCP) or knuckle joint.

flexion and extension From the "anatomic position" of the body (standing with the feet forward, the arms at the sides, and the palms forward), motions of the distal (distant) body segments toward the front, such as bending forward or making a fist with the fingers, are *flexion* motions. Motions backward, such as straightening a bent elbow or arching the back, are *extension* motions.

flexure contracture Inability to completely straighten (extend) a joint.

foramina See nerve root.

fusion or arthrodesis A "solid" joint that no longer moves. Fusion can result from an inherited abnormality, an injury, or surgery designed to obliterate that joint.

Golgi tendon apparatus Receptors in tendons that can sense stretch.

greater trochanter Bony prominence at the outer top of the thigh bone on which the abductor muscles of the hip insert.

hanging hip operation Lengthening of the tendons of the major muscle groups about the hip in order to decrease their force of contraction and thus lower the overall force on the hip joint.

hematoma A blood clot.

hematopoietic cells Cells of the red marrow that form blood cells.

humeral head and glenoid (glenohumeral joint) The ball (humeral head or upper end of the arm bone) and socket (glenoid) of the shoulder blade make up what most people refer to as the "shoulder joint." Shoulder motion technically also includes the motion of the shoulder blade on the chest wall.

hyaluronate A very large molecule containing repetitive sugars linked together and joined with protein. The molecule's primary function is presumably to lubricate soft tissues as they glide over each other.

hyperextension Overstraightening (*i.e.,* beyond anatomically straight).

hypertrophy Growing larger (*e.g.,* bony hypertrophy refers to additional bone formation beyond the limits of normal).

idiopathic Of unknown cause.

ilium Large flat bone that makes up the sides of the pelvis. We put our hands over the top of them when we "have our hands on our hips." The hip joint is really near the bottom of the pelvis and is difficult to feel.

infection A form of inflammation usually caused by an infectious agent such as bacteria or virus.

inflammation The process by which our bodies respond to injury. Inflammation is a cellularly mediated "clean-up and repair" operation. For example, when we puncture our finger with a wooden splinter, the tissue around the splinter is invaded by inflammatory cells that break down the tissue, forming pus. Meanwhile, this surrounding tissue is invaded by small blood vessels, making it appear red and possibly causing local heat as well. As soon as the splinter has been removed and the pus drained away, the cells associated with the blood vessels repair the tissues, and the inflammatory process subsides. Pus is not an essential component of the inflammatory process, which sometimes may be characterized only by increased vascularity and swelling (edema) of the involved tissues.

intercondylar femoral groove See patellofemoral joint.

internal and external rotation The rotation of a body segment as viewed from above the body. If the arm is held at the side and the elbow is bent, bringing one's forearm across the chest is *internal rotation* of the arm. *External rotation* of the arm brings the forearm out to one's side.

interphalangeal joints Joints of the fingers. *See* finger joints.

intervertebral foramen The bony channel through which the nerve roots exit the spinal column to form nerves.

intramembranous and endochondral bone formation Bone can be formed either from tissue, for example, the fibrous layer or periosteum, which cloaks the shaft of a bone (*intramembranous bone formation*), or from a cartilaginous mold or growth plate (*endochondral bone formation*).

intrinsic and extrinsic muscles of the hand *Intrinsic muscles* of the hand are those which originate in the hand itself. These are the interossei, lumbricals, and small muscles particular to the thumb and small finger. All other muscles that can move the fingers and thumb originate in the forearm or just above the elbow and are called the *extrinsic muscles* of the hand.

in vitro Dead material or parts of bodies, including parts kept alive artificially.

in vivo Living material within a living organism.

IVP and flat plate of the abdomen *IVP* is a special x-ray view taken after an injection of radiopaque dye, which makes the kidneys and urinary collecting system visible radiographically. A *flat plate of the abdomen* is a routine x-ray view of the belly.

kyphosis Hump- or hunchback.

laminectomy Surgical removal of part of the bony posterior elements of the spine in order to surgically reveal the spinal cord or nerve roots.

lateral *See* medial and lateral.

ligamenta nuchae Dense fibrous bands that run between the cervical spinous processes and the back of the skull strengthening the cervical area.

ligamentum teres A vascular band from the center of the hip joint socket to the center of the femoral head.

lordosis Swayback deformity.

lumbosacral facet Small, vertically oriented intervertebral joints between the posterior portions of the lowest lumbar vertebrae (L5) and the sacrum (pelvis). This is where the spine meets the pelvis, and, because this region is subject to great stress from the upright posture, these facet joints are subject to frequent mechanically induced problems.

malleolus The bony prominence on the inside or outside of the ankle.

medial and lateral *Medial* is toward the center line of the body; *lateral* is away from the center line.

mesenchymal cells Cells capable of differentiation into those that create fibrous connective tissue (fibroblasts), cartilage (chondroblasts), or bone (osteoblasts).

metacarpophalangeal joint *See* finger joints.

metaphyseal dysplasia Growth abnormality at the ends of bones, believed to be congenital in origin.

metaphysis The end of the bone that includes the bony parts of the joint, the growth plate (epiphysis), and the supporting trabecular bone structure, which subsequently opens up to form the marrow cavity. The central part of the bone encompassing the shaft and marrow cavity is called the diaphysis.

metastatic Cancer that has spread to beyond its place of origin other than by direct expansion of the primary tumor.

metatarsus adductus Turning inward of the toes and the forepart of the foot.

MMPI The Minnesota Multiphasic Personality Inventory is a psychological test.

muscular dystrophy A slow, progressive weakness in muscles that occurs as a consequence of some genetically inherited trait. This condition usually begins up about the hips and causes weakness in the lower extremities.

myelodysplasia A congenital abnormality involving failure of the spinal tube to close *in utero*. In severe cases the child is born with the spinal contents in a sac on its back instead of enclosed within the spinal canal. This is usually associated with some paralysis in the lower extremities.

myelogram Roentgenogram taken after radiopaque dye has been injected into the spinal canal so that soft-tissue impingements on the spinal cord and nerve roots can be visualized radiographically.

navicular Small bone of the midfoot, just in front of the talus.

neck of the femur The top of the thigh bone which enters the hip joint. The most upper part of the bone is thus within the hip joint and is not surrounded by vascularized periosteum. This explains the difficulties in the healing of this fracture. Blood supply to the upper fragment comes in mostly from below, and the fracture fragments can be rendered avascular (without any blood supply).

neoplasm Cancer.

nerve root These are filaments of spinal neural tissue coming off the spinal cord to form nerves that pass into the parts of the body they serve. Because the spinal cord is surrounded by the bone of the vertebral column, there are holes in the bone (foramina) for the nerve roots to pass through.

nonunion *See* delayed union and nonunion.

open fracture A fracture of bone that communicates to the outside through a hole or break in the overlaying skin.

osteoarthrosis Deterioration of a joint with loss of the articular cartilage-bearing surface associated with new-bone formation. Also called osteoarthritis or degenerative joint disease.

osteochondral fractures Fracture involving a piece of the articular cartilage surface of a joint or its underlying bony bed. These fractures are usually small and difficult to diagnose since they are not usually visible on x-ray film.

osteoclasis Removal of bone. It is carried out by special cells (osteoclasts).

osteomyelitis Infection in bone.

osteonecrosis Bone death. In a living subject, dead bone is slowly removed and slowly replaced. The removal and replacement phases overlap, and it is during this period that the structural integrity of the healing bony segment is impaired. Thus collapse and fracture through or around a healing osteonecrotic segment are common.

osteoporosis Thinned bones, that is, less bone mass than normal.

osteotomy The realignment of a bone by a surgically induced fracture.

patella Kneecap.

patellofemoral joint The joint between the kneecap (*patella*) and the distal end of the thigh bone (*femur*). The indentation in the end of the femur in which the kneecap tracks is called the intercondylar femoral groove.

periosteum Vascularized fibrous tissue that surrounds the shafts of the long bones. It provides intramembranous bone formation (for growth and repair) and vascularity for the outer aspects of the bony shaft.

phlebitis Inflammation of veins. It is associated with the formation of clots in these veins (thrombophlebitis) which can break off and lodge in vital structures. This is the major cause of pulmonary embolism.

plantar flexion To bring the foot down, that is, toe pointing toward the floor.

plasma exudate The liquid phase of blood (minus its cells) which has seeped out of the blood vessels and into the tissues.

prostatitis Inflammation of the prostate gland.

proteoglycan Large molecules containing sugars and proteins that are found in high abundance in cartilage. The sulfated ones have sulfur attached.

proximal and distal *Proximal* is the direction toward the center of the body, and *distal* is the direction away from the center of the body. For example, the foot is at the distal end of the leg.

proximal interphalangeal joint *See* finger joints.

psychic potentiation Imagined increase in the severity of symptoms. If it is unconscious, the patient is not aware that he is making the symptoms seem far worse than they really are.

pulmonary embolism Blood clots in the body that break off and enter the circulation are filtered out by the small blood vessels of the lungs. This functionally inactivates the section of the lungs involved. Pulmonary embolism, if it is massive enough, can cause instant death from asphyxiation.

pyrophosphate Chemical form of one of the ingredients of the substance that calcifies bone.

quadriceps femoris Part of the large quadriceps muscle that makes up the front part of the thigh and straightens the knee. Its tendon contains the patella.

radial and ulnar sides of the hand The *radial side* of the hand is the side of the hand that articulates, via the wrist, with the radius; that is, it is the side of the hand the thumb is on. The *ulnar side* of the hand articulates, via the wrist, with the ulna bone of the forearm. It is the side of the hand the ring and small fingers are on.

recurvatum of the knee Standing with the knee hyperstraight so that the knee appears to be concave from the front.

referred pain Awareness of a discomfort removed from the actual pathology. Besides sciatica and cervical radiculitis, another example is a gallbladder attack, which the patient sometimes feels only under the right shoulder blade. The basis of the phenomenon is shared nerve distribution. For example, the gallbladder sits right under the diaphragm, which is innervated by the same nerve roots as the region just under the shoulder blade. Irritation of the diaphragm is perceived as irritation of the nerve root but in another location (the shoulder blade) served by the same nerve root.

reflex testing Elicitation of the deep tendon reflexes by striking the tendon of a muscle, usually with a rubber hammer. This excites the muscle to contract and create an involuntary motion or jerk. The "knee jerk" and "ankle jerk" are reflexes.

retrocecal appendicitis Inflammation of the appendix when it is positioned deep in the abdomen, along its posterior wall, and thus just forward of the spine. The patient perceives back rather than belly pain.

scaphoid A wrist bone. Its blood supply comes in from only one end, and thus fracture through the middle of the bone can deprive the other end of its blood supply.

sciatica Pain in the lower extremity caused by pressure on or irritation of nerve roots in the lower spine.

scoliosis Curved spine as viewed from the front to back.

spinal stenosis Narrowing of the spinal canal.

spondylosis Osteoarthrosis of the spine.

stress fractures Fracture of bone caused by repetitive trauma rather than by significant injury. Such fractures do not show up on routine radiographic examination.

stress sparing When a rigid and less rigid member both share a load, the stiff member will take almost all of it, sparing the less stiff member. An example is a metal plate screwed firmly onto a bone. The plate is much stiffer and "stress spares" the underlying bone.

subchondral bone The bony bed upon which the articular cartilage of a joint rests. It is composed of a subchondral plate supported by interconnected trabecular bony struts.

subcutaneous Just under the skin.

subdeltoid bursitis Wherever a muscle passes over a bony prominence, nature forms a lubricating sac, or bursa, between the two. Inflammation of this sac, or bursitis, can occur. The subdeltoid bursa is the one on the outer (lateral) aspect of the shoulder.

subluxation A partial disruption of the integrity of a joint allowing the joint to momentarily slip partially out of place. Subluxations always self-reduce. If the joint stays completely out of its socket, it is a dislocation. *Subluxed* generally means a joint that is permanently partially out of its socket.

synovitis Inflammation of the synovium, or inner lining, of a joint.

talus The foot bone that sits above the heel bone and articulates with the leg bones to form the ankle joint.

tenosynovitis Inflammation of the sheath that encloses some tendons.

trabecular bone See cancellous bone.

ulnar side of the hand See radial and ulnar sides of the hand.

unilateral Affecting only one side.

valgus See varus and valgus.

varus and valgus *Varus* is an angle that a body segment makes toward the center line of the body. *Valgus* is the opposite. "Bowlegs" have varus knees. "Knock-knees" are valgus knees.

varus or inversion of the heel A deformity in which the heel is turned inward so that the patient tends to walk on the outside of his foot.

vasodilation Increase in diameter of blood vessels.

venous pressure Tissues require a blood supply, but it is also important for the blood, once oxygen and other nutrients have been removed from it, to flow away from the tissue. Otherwise, the tissue will remain congested and swelling will occur. If the swelling is severe enough, it may not be possible to effectively pump new blood into this area. The veins carry the blood away. Increased venous pressure is increased resistance to this outflow. The engorged veins, containing nerve endings in their walls, cause the pain associated with increases in venous pressure. If the venous pressure becomes high enough, blood circulation to that region will stop, and death of the tissue involved will occur.

ventral The front (anterior) of the body in the anatomic position.

vertebral numbering The vertebrae or backbones are grouped as neck (cervical), chest (thoracic), low back (lumbar), and pelvic (sacral). At the very bottom are the coccygeal (tail remnants). The vertebrae are numbered from the top so that C1 is the first cervical vertebra; C8, the eighth (and last) cervical vertebra; T12, the twelfth (and last) thoracic vertebra; and L5, the fifth (and last) lumbar vertebra. S1 is the top of the sacrum.

wallerian degeneration A specific term relating to degeneration of a nerve fiber following its transection or rupture.

Index

Index

The letter *f* after a page number indicates a figure; *t* following a page number indicates tabular material.

abductor pollicis brevis, testing of, 49
abductor pollicis longus tendon, inflammation of, 45–46, 47f
abscess
 in bone, 89
 of finger pulp, 55, 55f
 in joint, 90–91
acetabulum. *See* Hip
Achilles tendon, rupture of, 68
acromioclavicular joint, separation of, 67, 67f
acrylic cement in joint replacement, 109
active range of motion, 4
age, bone tumor and, 84–85
Allis' sign, 144f, 146
amputation in bone tumor, 86
angular deformity in physical examination, 5
angularity of lower extremity in infant, 137, 139–140, 140f
ankle
 deformity of, gait and, 151–152, 153f, 154, 157
 position of, in newborn, 137
annulus fibrosus, rupture of, 115–116
antalgic gait, 150
anteversion of femur, 138–139, 138f
antibiotics
 in hand infection, 53–55
 in joint infection, 90–91
 in osteomyelitis, 88–89
arteriography in tumor diagnosis, 79, 81f

arthritis
 arthrodesis in, 106–107, 107f
 definition of, 98–99
 diagnosis of, 99, 100f
 joint replacement in, 107–111, 108f
 juvenile, limp and, 158–159
 osteotomy contraindications in, 106
 synovectomy in, 103–104
 treatment of, 101, 103
arthrodesis in joint disease, 106–107, 107f
arthroplasty, 107–111, 108f
arthroscopy of knee, 71
arthrosis
 arthrodesis in, 106–107, 107f
 cervical, 61
 definition of, 98–100
 diagnosis of, 99–101, 102f
 after joint infection, 90
 joint replacement in, 107–111, 108f
 nodal, 101
 osteotomy in, 104, 105f, 106
 in spondylosis, 118–119
 synovectomy in, 103–104
 treatment of, 101, 103
aspirin
 in arthritis, 101
 in back pain, 127
athletic injury. *See* Sports injury
atlas, anatomy of, 57, 58f
axis, anatomy of, 57, 58f
axon, damage of, 47
axonotmesis, 47

183

Index

back-kneeing, 151–152
back pain, 113–127
　management of, 126–127
　physical examination in, 5
　psychological factors in, 126
　from pulled muscle, 113–114, 115f
　from ruptured disc, 114–121, 116f, 121f
　from sciatica, 114–115, 116f, 117, 119
　from spinal stenosis, 123f, 124, 126
　from spondylolisthesis, 124, 125f
　from spondylolysis, 124
　from spondylosis, 117–119, 118f, 123f
Barlow's test, 144f, 145
baseball finger, 43–44, 45f
Bennett's fracture, 53, 54f
biceps muscle, rupture of, 68
biomechanics
　in fracture, 9–10, 10f–11f
　of joint, 96–97, 94f–95f, 97f–98f, 104
　of sports injury, 63–66, 65f
biopsy in bone tumor diagnosis, 85
bite of hand, 42
blood loss in fracture, 21
blood supply in bone healing, 19–20
body weight, joint forces and, 63–64
bone. *See also specific bone, e.g.,* Femur; Tibia
　cancellous. *See also* Bone, trabecular
　　healing of, 18–19
　cortical, 77
　　healing of, 18–19
　embryology of, 131, 132f, 133–134, 134f–135f, 136
　fracture of. *See* Fracture
　growth of, 131, 132f, 133–134, 134f–135f, 136
　in infant, 136–137, 137f
　healing of. *See* Fracture, healing of
　infection of. *See* Osteomyelitis
　remodeling of
　　in growth, 131, 133
　　in hip dislocation, 148

　trabecular, 77, 96, 97f–98f. *See also* Bone, cancellous
　tumor of. *See* Tumor
bone cement in joint replacement, 109
bone scan in tumor diagnosis, 79, 81f
bony end plate, 96
boutonniere deformity, 42–43, 44f
bowing
　of femur, 139–140, 140f
　of tibia in child, 139–140, 140f
brace in scoliosis, 164
breech presentation, hip dislocation and, 142
bursitis
　of shoulder, 5
　in sports injury, 70

callus in bone healing, 14–17, 17f
cancellous bone. *See also* Trabecular bone
　healing of, 18–19
carpal tunnel syndrome, 48–49, 48f
cartilage
　articular, physiology of, 94–97, 94f–95f
　in bone growth, 131, 132f, 133
　in bone healing, 15–16, 17f
　fibrillation of, 96–97
cast
　in fracture, 20
　in metatarsus adductus, 141
cauda equina, impingement on, 123f, 124, 126
cement in joint replacement, 109
cerebral palsy, limping in, 155
cervical radiculitis, 60–61
cervical spine. *See also* Neck
　anatomy of, 57–58, 58f
　dislocation of, 60
　fracture of, 60
Charcot-Marie-Tooth disease, 157
charley horse, 69
Charnley joint replacement, 108–109

chemotherapy in bone tumor, 86
children. *See* Pediatric patients
chondrocytes, 97
chondrosarcoma, 86
chymopapain in ruptured disc, 120–121
claudication, spinal, 123f, 124, 126
clawed toes, 154
clenched-fist injury, 42
clubfoot, 141–142
coach's finger, 52–53, 53f
collagen, 94–95, 94f
Colles' fracture, reduction of, 25f
common extensor tendon, injury of, 69–70
computed tomography
  in back pain, 120, 122f–123f
  in tumor diagnosis, 79, 80f
congenital conditions
  of foot, 140–142
  of hip, 142–143, 144f, 145–146, 147f, 148
  limp and, 157
  of neck, 59
  rotational variations, 137–140, 138f, 140f
contracture in arthritis, 101
corset in back pain, 124, 127
cortical bone, 77
  healing of, 18–19
creeping substitution in bone healing, 19
crepitus in fracture, 12
cross-linking of collagen, 94, 94f
crush injury of hand, 44–45, 46f
cubital tunnel syndrome, 49–50
curvature of spine. *See* Scoliosis
cutting cones in bone healing, 14, 14f

  in fracture healing, 30
  in physical examination, 5
delayed union, 13
  causes of, 19–20
de Quervain's tenosynovitis, 45–46, 47f
diaphyseal fracture, 29–30
  in sports, 72
diaphysis in bone growth, 134, 134f–135f
disc, intervertebral
  rupture of, 61, 114–121, 116f, 121f, 123f
  space in, 122f–123f
dislocation
  of cervical spine, 60
  clinical features of, 10–12
  definition of, 10
  diagnosis of, 10–12, 31–32
  of elbow, 32
  emergency management of, 22
  of hip. *See* Hip, dislocation of
  in joint infection, 90
  of knee, 32
  of patellofemoral joint, 32
  radiographic examination of, 12–13, 13f
  recurrent, of shoulder, 31–32
  rehabilitation after, 33
  of shoulder, 30–32
distal interphalangeal joint, 42–43, 44f
  mallet deformity of, 43–44, 45f
dorsiflexion of foot, 154
drop foot
  in Charcot-Marie-Tooth disease, 157
  gait and, 151, 154
dropped finger, 43–44, 45f

débridement in osteomyelitis, 89–90
deformity. *See also* Congenital conditions
  in dislocation, 12
  in fracture, 12

edema in hand injury, 36
effusion, joint, 73–74, 99
  hip, 156
  in infection, 90
  in physical examination, 4

186 Index

elbow
  cubital tunnel syndrome at, 49–50
  dislocation of, 32
  fracture of, 31
  position of, in newborn, 136
  tendonitis of, 69–70
embryology of bone, 131, 132f, 133–134, 134f–135f, 136
emergency management of fracture, 21–22
endochondral ossification, 15, 131, 132f, 133–134, 134f
endochondromatosis, 84
epiphysis
  in bone growth, 132f, 133–134, 134f
  femoral, slipped, 157
  injury to, 29, 30f
  necrosis of, 155–156
equinus deformity of foot
  gait and, 151, 153f
  varus, 141–142
Ewing's sarcoma, 86
examination. See Physical examination; Radiographic examination
exercise
  in back pain, 127
  in clubfoot, 141–142
  in congenital conditions, 136
  in hip rotation, 139
  in metatarsus adductus, 141
extensor pollicis brevis tendon, inflammation of, 45–46, 47f
extensor retinaculum of wrist, 44–45, 46f
extensor tendon, injury of, 42, 43f
external fixation of fracture, 26
extracompartmental bone tumor, 84

fatigue fracture. See Stress fracture
felon, 55, 55f
femur. See also Hip
  anteversion of, 138–139, 138f
  bowing of, 139–140, 140f

epiphysis of, slipped, 157
fracture of, 23f, 28, 28f
head of, osteonecrosis of, 155–156
osteosarcoma of, 77, 78f, 80f–82f
fetus. See also Intrauterine position
  bone development in, 131, 132f, 133–134, 134f–135f, 136
fibrillation of cartilage, 96–97
fibrosarcoma, 86
finger. See Hand
fingernail, infection around, 54f, 55
Finkelstein test, 45–46, 47f
flexor digitorum profundus tendon, examination of, 38, 38f
flexor digitorum superficialis tendon, examination of, 38–39, 38f–39f
flexor tendon, injury of, 40–42, 41f
flexor tendon sheath, infection of, 55
foot
  deformity of, gait and, 151–152, 153f, 154, 157
  dorsiflexion of, 154
  in gait, 150
  plantar-flexed, 141–142
  position of, in newborn, 137
  toeing-in of, 139
  turning-in of, 140–141
football, knee injury in, 70–71
footprint in metatarsus adductus, 141
force. See also Biomechanics
  on joint, 93–97, 94f–95f, 97f–98f
  redistribution of, with osteotomy, 104, 105f
forearm, fracture of, 30
fracture
  arthrosis and, 100
  biomechanics of, 9–10, 10f–11f
  causes of, 9–10, 11f, 65–66, 65f
  of cervical spine, 60
  clinical features of, 10–12
  closed, 20
  definition of, 9
  diagnosis of, 10–12
  diaphyseal, 29–30
    in sports, 72
  of elbow, 31

epiphyseal, 29, 30f
of forearm, 30
of hand, 50–53, 50f–54f
healing of, 13–20
    factors affecting, 19–20
    inflammatory phase, 15, 16f
    by primary intention, 14, 14f
    proliferative phase, 15–16, 17f
    prolonged, 13
    remodeling phase, 17–19, 18f
    by secondary intention, 14–19, 14f, 16f–18f
    stress in, 27
immobilization of, 26–28, 27f–28f
infection in, 20, 28–29
management of, 20–28
    definitive, 22–24, 23f–25f
    emergency, 21–22
    immobilization in, 26–28, 27f–28f
open, 20, 28–29
pathological, 10, 20, 79, 80
in pediatric patients, 29–31, 30f
radiographic examination of, 12–13
reduction of, 23–24, 23f–25f, 27
rehabilitation after, 32–33
in sports, 72–73
stress, 72–73
    causes of, 10
    limp and, 157
    through pars articularis, 124
    in sports, 72–73
functional loss in fracture, 12
fusion
    in joint disease, 106–107, 107f
    of spine
        cervical, 59
        in intervertebral disc disease, 119
        in scoliosis, 163

gait
    components of, 150–152, 151f–153f

evaluation of, 158
Galleazzi's sign, 144f, 145–146
genu valgum, 139–140, 140f
genu varum, 139–140, 140f
girdle in back pain, 124, 127
gluteus maximus limp, 150–151, 152f
gluteus medius limp, 150, 151f
gold in arthritis, 101
Golgi apparatus in muscle injury, 68
gout vs. joint infection, 90
granulation tissue in bone healing, 14, 17f
greater trochanter advancement, 104, 105f
gross deformity in physical examination, 5
ground substance, 94–95
growth of bone, 131, 132f, 133–134, 134f–135f, 136
    arrest of, 30
    in infant, 136–137, 137f
growth plate, injury to, 29, 30f

hand. *See also* Wrist
    functions of, 35
    infection in, 53–55, 54f–55f
    injury of, 35–55
        boutonniere deformity, 42–43, 44f
        carpal tunnel syndrome, 48–49, 48f
        crush, 44–45, 46f
        cubital tunnel syndrome, 49–50
        de Quervain's tenosynovitis, 45–46, 47f
        dislocation in, 42–43, 53f
        examination in, 36–40, 37f–40f
        extensor tendon, 42, 43f
        flexor tendon, 40–42, 41f
        fracture in, 50–53, 50f–54f
        history in, 36
        human bite, 42
        mallet deformity, 43–44, 45f
        nerve, 39–40, 39f–40f, 46–47
        treatment goals in, 35
        trigger finger, 46–47

healing
  of fracture. See Fracture, healing of
  of ligament, 66
heat in back pain, 127
heel cord, rupture of, 68
heel pain, limp and, 158
heel strike, 150
hematoma in fracture, 15, 16f–17f
hemorrhage, control of, in fracture, 21
hip
  dislocation of, 13f
    diagnosis of, 144f, 145–146
    etiology of, 142–143
    limping in, 155
    pathomechanics of, 143, 144f, 145
    treatment of, 148
    x-ray finding in, 146, 147f, 148
  hanging, in arthrosis, 104, 106
  motion of, in gait, 150–151, 151f
  osteotomy of, 106
  position of, in newborn, 136
  replacement of, 108–111, 108f
  rotation of, 138–139, 138f
history, medical, 3–4
  in hand injury, 36
  in limping child, 154–158
hormones
  in bone growth, 133, 136
  in hip dislocation, 143
hyaluronic acid, 96

immunosuppressive therapy in arthritis, 101
implant, joint, 107–111, 108f
infant. See also Congenital conditions; Newborn
  bone development in, 136–137, 137f
infection
  of bone. See Osteomyelitis
  in fracture, 20, 28–29
  in hand, 53–55, 54f–55f
  in hand bite injury, 42

hematogenous, 87
  in joint, 4, 74, 90–91
  in joint replacement, 111
inflammation of synovial membrane, 96–97
inflammatory phase in bone healing, 15, 16f
inflammatory response in ruptured disc, 117
injury. See specific injury, e.g., Dislocation; Fracture; specific body part, e.g., Knee
interferon in osteosarcoma, 86–87
internal fixation in fracture, 26–27, 27f
intervertebral disc
  rupture of, 61, 114–121, 116f, 121f, 123f
  space in, 122f–123f
intracompartmental bone tumor, 84
intramedullary nailing, 27–28, 28f
intramembranous ossification, 131, 133, 135f
intrauterine position
  in hip dislocation, 142–143
  in hip rotation, 139
  in metatarsus adductus, 140
  normal joint positions and, 136–137
  in tibial torsion, 139
intrinsic-plus position, 52, 52f
involucrum in osteomyelitis, 88, 88f

jogging, stress fracture in, 72–73
joint. See also specific joint
  dislocation of. See Dislocation
  effusion in, 4, 99
    traumatic, 73–74
  forces acting on, 63–66, 64f
  infection in, 4, 90–91
  inflammation of. See Arthritis; Arthrosis
  injury of. See Dislocation; Sprain; Strain
  pathology of, 96–97

physiology of, 93–97, 94f–95f, 97f–98f
radiographic examination of, in children, 6
range of motion of, 4–5
 in newborn, 136
replacement of, 107–111, 108f
joint capsule
 biomechanics of, 64
 physiology of, 95–96
jumper's knee, 157

Klippel-Feil syndrome, 59
Knavel's signs, 55
knee
 arthrodesis of, 107f
 arthrosis of, 103f
 biomechanics of, 64–65
 dislocation of, 32
 effusion on, 74
 examination of, 5, 159
 fracture of, 72
 hyperextension of, 151–152
 jumper's, 157
 malposition of, 139–140, 140f
 meniscus of, tearing of, 70–72, 71f
 motion of, in gait, 151–152, 153f, 154
 osteotomy of, 106
 pain in, 155, 159
 position of, in newborn, 136–137
 in slipped capital femoral epiphysis, 157
knock-knees, 139–140, 140f
 dislocation and, 32
knuckles, injury of, 42
kyphosis in scoliosis, 163

laboratory study of limping child, 159
Lasègue's sign, 119
Legg-Calvé-Perthes disease, 155–156

leg raising, back pain and, 119
length of limb, evaluation of, 158
lifting, back pain and, 113–114, 115f
ligament
 biomechanics of, 64
 to neck, injury to, 60
 radiographic examination of, 6
 sprain of, 66–69, 67f
ligamentum teres, occlusion of, 156
limb length, evaluation of, 158
limping child, 149–159
 gait components and, 150–152, 151f–153f
 laboratory studies of, 159
 medical history and, 154–158
 physical examination of, 158–159
load characteristics in fracture, 9
long bone, growth of, 131, 132f, 133–134, 134f–135f
loose body in knee, 72
loosening of joint replacement, 109–111
lordosis
 appearance of, in infant, 136–137, 137f
 in scoliosis, 163
low back pain. See Back pain
lower extremity, rotational deformity of, 137–140, 138f, 140f
lubrication in joint, 96
lung, bone metastasis from, 85–86
lymphoma, treatment of, 86

McMurray's test, 71
malignancy. See Tumor
malleolus in tibial rotation, 139
mallet deformity, 43–44, 45f
manipulation of fracture, 24, 25f
medial tibial torsion, 139
median nerve
 compression of, 48–49, 48f
 testing of, 39–40, 40f, 49
medical history, 3–4
 in hand injury, 36
 in limping child, 154–158

meniscectomy, 72
meniscus of knee, tearing of, 70–72, 71f
mesenchymal cells
  in bone growth, 131, 132f
  in bone healing, 15
metacarpal joint of thumb, fracture of, 53, 54f
metaphysis
  in bone growth, 134, 134f
  infection of, 90
metastasis to bone, 79, 81, 84–85, 84t
metatarsus adductus, 140–141
methotrexate in arthritis, 101
methyl methacrylate in joint replacement, 109
muscle
  in back, strain of, 126–127
  fatigue of, in sports injury, 65–66, 72–73
  forces produced by, 63–66, 64f
  pulling of, 68
  spasm of, 114, 115f
    in back pain, 113–114, 115f
    in fracture, 22
  tearing of, 68–69
    back pain and, 113–114, 115f
myelodysplasia, gait in, 154
myelography
  in back pain, 119–120, 120f–121f
myeloma, treatment of, 86

nail, intramedullary, 27–28, 28f
neck. *See also* Cervical spine
  congenital disorders of, 59
  dislocation of, 60
  fracture of, 60
  injury of, examination of, 58
  radiculitis of, 60–61
  soft-tissue injury of, 59–60
necrosis
  in joint infection, 91
  in osteomyelitis, 87–90, 88f
needle biopsy in bone tumor diagnosis, 85

neonate. *See* Newborn
nerve in hand
  injury to, 47–50, 48f
  testing of, 39–40, 39f–40f
neurapraxia, 47
neurotmesis, 47
newborn. *See also* Congenital conditions
  bone development in, 131, 132f, 133–134, 134f–135f, 136
nodal osteoarthrosis, 101
"no man's land" in finger, 40, 41f
nonsteroidal anti-inflammatory agents
  in arthritis, 101
  in arthrosis, 103
nonunion, 13
  causes of, 19–20

odontoid, anatomy of, 57, 58f
Ollier's disease, 84
onlay plate in fracture, 26, 27f
Ortolani's sign, 144f, 145–146
Osgood-Schlatter disease, 157
ossification, 131, 132f, 133–134, 134f
osteoarthrosis. *See* Arthrosis
osteoblasts in bone healing, 14f, 15, 17
osteochondral fracture in sports, 72
osteochondritis dissecans, 72
osteoclasts in bone healing, 14f, 17
osteolysis in osteomyelitis, 87–88
osteomyelitis, 87–91
  acute, 87
  causes of, 87
  chronic, 87–88, 88f
  diagnosis of, 77–79, 78f, 80f–82f, 87
  limping in, 155, 159
  recurrence of, 89
osteonecrosis
  in dislocation, 10
  of femoral head, 155–156
osteoporosis, fracture in, 9–10

osteosarcoma, 84
  treatment of, 86–87
  x-ray of, 77, 78f, 80f–82f
osteotomy
  in arthrosis, 104, 105f, 106
  in hip dislocation, 148

Paget's disease, 84
pain
  in back. *See* Back pain
  in dislocation, 11
  in fracture, 11
  in heel, 158
  in joint, 99, 101, 104, 106
  in limp, 154–155
  in medical history, 3
  referred, 3
    in limp, 154–155
    in sciatica, 117
palpation in physical examination, 4
paronychia, 54f, 55
pars articularis, fracture through, 124, 124f
passive range of motion, 4–5
patella, tendonitis of, 157
patellofemoral joint. *See also* Knee
  dislocation of, 32
  examination of, 5
pathological fracture, 10, 20, 79, 80
pediatric patients
  bone formation in, 131, 132f, 133–134, 134f–135f, 136
  foot problems in, 140–142
  fracture in, 29–31, 30f
  hip dislocation in, 142–143, 144f, 145–146, 147f, 148
  limping in. *See* Limping child
  normal infant development, 136–137
  rotational variation in, 137–140, 138f, 140f
  scoliosis in. *See* Scoliosis
  x-ray examination of, 6
pelvis, motion of, in gait, 150–151, 151f

penicillamine in arthritis, 101
perichondrium, 133
periosteum
  in bone growth, 131, 133, 134f–135f
  in bone healing, 15–16, 16f
Perthes' disease, 155–156
phalanx, fracture of, 50f, 52
Phalen's test, 49
physical examination, 4–5
  in hand injury, 36–40, 37f–40f
  in limp, 158–159
  of neck, 61
  in rotational deformity, 138
  in ruptured disc, 117
  in scoliosis, 163, 164f
physical therapy in joint disease, 103
pin in fracture reduction, 24, 26
plantaris tendon, rupture of, 68
primary intention in bone healing, 14
proliferative phase in bone healing, 15–16, 17f
prosthesis, joint, 107–111, 108f
proteoglycans, 94–95, 95f, 100
proximal interphalangeal joint
  flexion contracture of, 42–43, 44f
  fracture-dislocation of, 52–53, 53f
psychological factors in back pain, 126
pulley in hand, 40, 41f
pulmonary function in scoliosis, 163
pyarthrosis, 90–91
pyrophosphate uptake in tumor diagnosis, 79, 81f

quadriceps femoris limp, 152, 153f

radial nerve, testing of, 39–40, 40f
radiographic examination, 5–6. *See also* X-ray
  in dislocation, 12–13, 13f

radiographic examination (continued)
  in fracture, 12–13
  of neck, 58
radiotherapy in bone tumor, 86
range of motion
  in newborn, 136
  in physical examination, 4–5
recurvatum, knee, 151–152
reduction of fracture, 23–24, 23f–25f, 27
  in hand, 50, 50f–51f
referred pain, 3
  in limp, 154–155
  in sciatica, 117
rehabilitation
  in dislocation, 33
  in fracture, 32–33
remodeling of bone
  in growth, 131, 133, 135f
  in healing, 17–19, 18f
  in hip dislocation, 148
replacement of joint, 107–111, 108f
reserve curve, appearance of, in infant, 136–137, 137f
restraint in hip dislocation, 148
revision of joint replacement, 110
rheumatoid arthritis
  pathology of, 100f
  treatment of, 101, 103
ribs, scoliosis and, 162–163, 162f, 164f
rotation of lower extremity in infant, 137–140, 138f, 140f
running, normal, 149
rupture
  of intervertebral disc, 61, 114–121, 116f, 121f, 123f
  of muscle, 68–69
  of tendon, 67–69

Salter-Harris classification, 29, 30f
scar in flexor tendon injury, 40–41, 41f
sciatica, 114–115, 116f, 117, 119

scoliosis, 161–165
  causes of, 161
  characteristics of, 161–163, 162f
  examination for, 163, 164f
  progression of, 164
  treatment of, 163–165, 164f
secondary intention in bone healing, 14–19, 14f, 16f, 17f–18f
sequestrum in osteomyelitis, 87–88, 88f
shock-absorbing mechanism
  in arthrosis, 100
  for joints, 64
shock in fracture, 21
shoe, corrective, in metatarsus adductus, 141
shoulder
  bursitis of, 5, 70
  dislocation of, 31–32
  sprain of, 67, 67f
sinus tract drainage in osteomyelitis, 88
skeletal traction in fracture, 26
skeleton
  development of, 136–137, 137f
  embryology of, 131, 132f, 133–134, 134f–135f, 136
skin traction in fracture, 26
sling in fracture, 26
slipped capital femoral epiphysis, 157
soft-tissue injury to neck, 59–60
spasm, muscular, 114, 115f
  in back pain, 124
  in fracture, 22
spinal canal, 122f–123f
  stenosis of, 123f, 124, 126
spinal claudication, 123f, 124, 126
spinal cord in scoliosis, 163
spinal root, compression of, 114–121, 116f
spine. See also Cervical spine; Vertebra
  curvature of
    abnormal. See Scoliosis
    in normal infant, 136, 137f

injury of, emergency management of, 22
pain in. See Back pain
splint
 in back pain, 124, 127
 of fracture, 21–22
  hand, 52
spondylolisthesis, 124, 125f
 in limping child, 157
spondylolysis, 124
spondylosis, 117–119, 118f, 123f
 cervical, 61
sports injury, 63–74
 biomechanics of, 63–66, 65f
 bursitis, 70
 fractures, 72–73
 joint effusion, 73–74
 knee meniscus, 70–72, 71f
 sprain, 66–69, 67f
 strain, 66–69, 67f
 tendonitis, 69–70
sprain in sport injury, 66–69, 67f
staging of bone tumor, 84, 84t
stair climbing with quadriceps limp, 152, 153f
stance, 150
stenosis, spinal, 123f, 124, 126
steroids in arthritis, 101
strain
 of back muscles, 126–127
 in sport injury, 66–69, 67f
stress
 in arthrosis, 99–100
 in bone healing, 18, 27
stress fracture
 causes of, 10
 limp and, 157–158
 through pars articularis, 124
 in sports, 72–73
stretching. See Exercise
subchondral plate, 96
supraspinatus tendon, bursitis from, 70
surgery
 in bone tumor, 86
 in joint disease, 103
 in ruptured disc, 117, 121

 in scoliosis, 164
suture of tendon, 68
swaddling, hip dislocation and, 143
swelling, physical examination of, 4
swing, 150
synovectomy in joint disease, 103–104
synovial. See Joint
synovial fluid, 96
 examination of, 159
synovial membrane
 inflammation of, 96–97
 physiology of, 96
 trauma to, 73–74
synovitis
 in arthrosis, 100–101
 in limping child, 156

talipes equinovarus, 141–142
talus in clubfoot, 141
technetium bone scan, 79, 81f
tenderness
 in fracture, 12
 in physical examination, 4
tendon
 of hand
  examination of, 36–39, 37f–38f
  infection of, 55
  injury of, 40–47, 41f, 43f–48f
  rupture of, 67–69
  suture of, 68
tendonitis
 patellar, 157
 in sports injury, 69–70
tennis elbow, 69–70
tenosynovitis of hand, 45–47, 47f
thorax, scoliosis and, 162–163, 162f, 164f
thumb
 fracture of, 53, 54f
 pain in, 45–46, 47f
 tenosynovitis of, 46–47
tibia
 bowing of
  in child, 139–140, 140f

tibia (*continued*)
  in newborn, 136
  rotation of, 138–139
    with metatarsus adductus, 141
  tubercle of
    advancement, 104, 105f
    avulsion of, 157
tidemark in joint, 94, 94f
Tinel's sign, 49
toe, clawed, 154
toeing in, 139
toeing off, 150
toe walking, 154
torticollis, 59
  with hip dislocation, 143
tourniquet in fracture, 21
trabecular bone, 77, 96, 97f–98f. See also Cancellous bone
traction in fracture, 21–22, 24, 24f, 26
transmalleolar axis, 139
trauma. *See specific type, e.g.,* Dislocation; Fracture
Trendelenburg gait, 150, 151f
trigger finger, 46–47
trigger thumb, 46–47
tuberculosis of bone, 87
tumor
  of bone, 79–87
    age and, 84–85
    classification of, 81, 83t, 84
    diagnosis of, 77–79, 78f, 80f–82f, 85
    metastatic, 79, 81, 84–85, 84t
    prognosis of, 85–86
    staging of, 84, 84t
    treatment of, 86–87
  in limping child, 155–157
two-point discrimination test, 39, 39f

ulnar nerve
  compression of, 49–50
  testing of, 39–40, 40f

valgus deformity of leg, 140, 140f
varus deformity of leg, 140, 140f
venous pressure
  in arthrosis, 103
  in joint pain, 99
  in osteomyelitis, 89
vertebra. *See also* Spine
  scoliosis and, 162–163, 162f
  slipping of, 124, 125f

walking. *See also* Gait
  normal, 149
  spinal claudication and, 126
water on the joint, 73–74
weight, body, joint forces and, 63–64
whiplash injury, 59–60
Wolff's law, 27
wrist. *See also* Hand
  extensor retinaculum of, 44–45, 46f
  fracture of, 25f
wryneck, 59
  with hip dislocation, 143

x-ray. *See also* Radiographic examination
  in hip dislocation, 146, 147f, 148
  of limping child, 159
  in tumor diagnosis, 77–79, 78f
  views for, 5